Every Day is New Again:
Understanding Dementia

I0415353

Acknowledgement:
I am grateful to Philip Curtis whose insight sent me in a
new direction and made this book possible.

IEP Press
Palm Springs, California
www.rcfe-ceu.com

ISBN: 978-1456346423
ISBN-10: 1456346423

Printed in the United States of America

Table of Contents

Preface

Unlike other dementia materials, this focuses less on the biological causes and effects, in favor of understanding the psychological and sociological impact. This information will have a direct impact on day to day interaction with dementia clients; and allow one to see the person inside the disease. While not dismissing the need for understanding the biological impact, there will be a small portion on neuro-anatomy. Understanding the basic operations of the brain will be tied to understanding behaviors, motivations, and emotions.

The evaluation section will assist the reader in understanding how the symptoms of dementia usually begin to manifest. Although the administration of evaluation assessments require years of training, this section provides an introduction to some of the screening tools utilized by professionals. Perhaps the most important part of any evaluation is gathering historical information from family and caregivers. Detailed data on the clients performance of Activities of Daily Living (ADLs) provides important diagnostic information. This is where a residential care facility can "shine" – in their methodical record keeping. Some suggested forms are provided.

A treatment and therapeutic section is provided for dementia and Alzheimer's in particular. Although similar, there is much more research about Alzheimer's and therefore unique and targeted therapies. Understanding which therapies work best for each stage of the Alzheimer's disease could guide decisions to hire or consult with a local therapist. This understanding could also guide decisions to accept offers from local agencies claiming to provide effective interventions for Alzheimer's clients.

The brief section on other dementia syndromes provides an introduction and overview to understanding the differences. Not all dementia is Alzheimer's, others manifest in different ways; progress at different rates; and require different interventions. This section will provide some vocabulary and understanding which may help during the intake family interview of dementia patients. Further, it will provide the starting point for further research.

A final section on environmental changes will provide increased safety for Alzheimer's clients. This section is brief but very important. The interventions listed here can save lives and reduce stress of both staff and clients.

The information and interventions contained within come from reliable sources. Each source is referenced in the text and each chapter ends with a complete "works cited" page allowing a deeper understanding of most topics.

07 November 2010

Chapter 1 - Neuro-Anatomy

Terminology

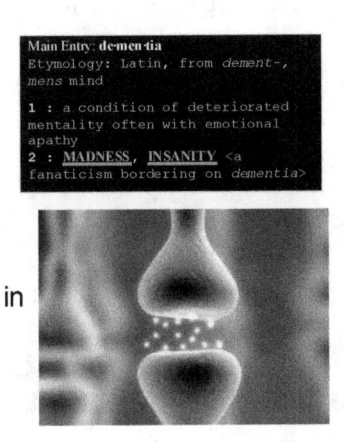

Main Entry: **de·men·tia**
Etymology: Latin, from *dement-*, *mens* mind

1 : a condition of deteriorated mentality often with emotional apathy
2 : <u>MADNESS</u>, <u>INSANITY</u> <a fanaticism bordering on *dementia*>

• Dementia

Acquired syndrome consisting of a decline in memory and other cognitive functions

In the common use of the word, dementia typically involves some type of insanity. When the word is used medically, the term dementia refers to an acquired syndrome consisting of a decline in memory and other cognitive or brain functions.

Source: (M. Pekker)
The Diagnostic Statistical Manual – 4th Edition (DSM-IV) requires the following in order to diagnose a person with dementia:

    A. The development of multiple cognitive deficits manifested by both:

      1. Memory impairment (impaired ability to learn new information or to recall previously learned information)

      2. One or more of the following cognitive disturbances:

- aphasia (language disturbance).
- apraxia (impaired ability to carry out motor activities despite intact motor function),
- agnosia (failure to recognize or identify objects despite intact sensory function),

- disturbance in executive functioning (i.e., planning, organizing, sequencing, abstracting).

B. The cognitive deficits in criteria A1 and A2 each cause significant impairment in social or occupational functioning and represent a significant decline from a previous level of functioning.

C. Focal neurological signs and symptoms (e.g., exaggeration of deep tendon reflexes, extensor plantar response, psuedobulbar palsy, gait abnormalities, weakness of an extremity) or laboratory evidence indicative of cerebrovascular disease (e.g., multiple infarctions involving cortex and underlying white matter) that are judged to be etiologically related to the disturbance.

D. The deficits do not occur exclusively during the course of a delirium.

Dementia's Definition

- Multiple Cognitive Deficits:
  - Memory dysfunction
    - especially new learning, prominent early symptom
  - At least one additional cognitive deficit
    - aphasia, apraxia, agnosia, or executive dysfunction
- Cognitive Disturbances:
  - Sufficiently severe to cause impairment of occupational or social functioning, and
  - Must represent decline from previous level of functioning

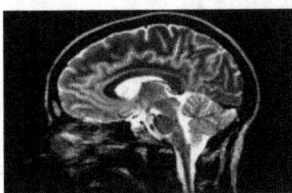
Source: (DementiaGuide)

It is important to compare dementia vs. Alzheimer's disease to realize the differences between the two conditions. Alzheimer's is the most common form of dementia marked by memory loss in older people. Dementia is the gradual loss of intellectual function. Alzheimer's statistics show the disease can strike a person as early as 45, while dementia generally takes hold after age 70. The most confused form of dementia is Multi-Infarct Dementia or MID. This condition also attacks the blood vessels in the brain. Both disorders require testing to determine the best course of treatment.

Dementia and Alzheimer's diseases are perhaps two of the most confusing diseases that exist in the realm of mental degradation in America today. There are a number of differences, however, that allow for those dealing with symptoms characteristic of these two diseases to become more informed.

Comparing the Two Diseases:
When comparing dementia vs. Alzheimer's disease it is very important to discuss the differences between the two diseases. Although they have many similarities, there are a number of differences that must be noted.

Alzheimer's disease is defined as a form of dementia characterized by the gradual loss of several important mental functions. It is perhaps the most common cause of dementia in older Americans, and goes beyond just normal forgetfulness, such as losing car keys or forgetting where one parked. Signs of Alzheimer's disease include memory loss that is much more severe and more serious, such as forgetting the names of one's children or perhaps where one lived for the last decade or two.

Another way to compare dementia vs. Alzheimer's disease is to realize that dementia is a medical term used to describe a number of conditions characterized by the gradual loss of intellectual function. Certain symptoms, as defined by the American Medical Association, of dementia include memory impairment, increased language difficulties, decreased motor skills, failure to recognized or identify objects, and disturbance of the ability to plan or think abstractly.

Yet another way to determine the differences of dementia vs. Alzheimer's disease is when the onset of the disease was first noticed. Of course, this is a very difficult thing since the progression of both is very gradual, and often there is no one point where someone can say, "Aha!" and know the disease has taken hold. Often the onset of Alzheimer's can occur as early as 45 years of age. General dementia, however, usually is noted later in life, perhaps in the 70 to 80 year range.

When looking at dementia vs. Alzheimer's disease, one type of dementia is often confused with Alzheimer's disease – Multi-Infarct Dementia or MID. MID is a common cause of dementia in the elderly and occurs when blood clots block small blood vessels in the brain and destroys brain tissue. Symptoms of MID, which are very similar to Alzheimer's disease, include confusion, problems with short term memory, wandering, and getting lost in familiar places, loss of bladder and bowel control, and emotional problems such as laughing or crying during inappropriate times.

Why Care about Dementia

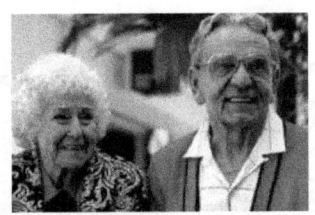

- "Graying" population
  - By 2030, may be 70 million elderly in United States (currently around 35 million)
- Current prevalence rates of dementia
  - 6-8% if older than 65
  - 30% if older than 80

Source: (Paul, 2005)

Why care about dementia? The average age of the US population is expected to increase dramatically in the coming decades. By 2030, there are expected to be 70 million elderly in the United States. (Defined as >65 years old). Because dementia is so prevalent in this population, a significant number can be expected to suffer from dementia. Current prevalence rates of dementia for those older than 65 range from 6 to 8 percent. For those older than 80, the rate is as high as 30%

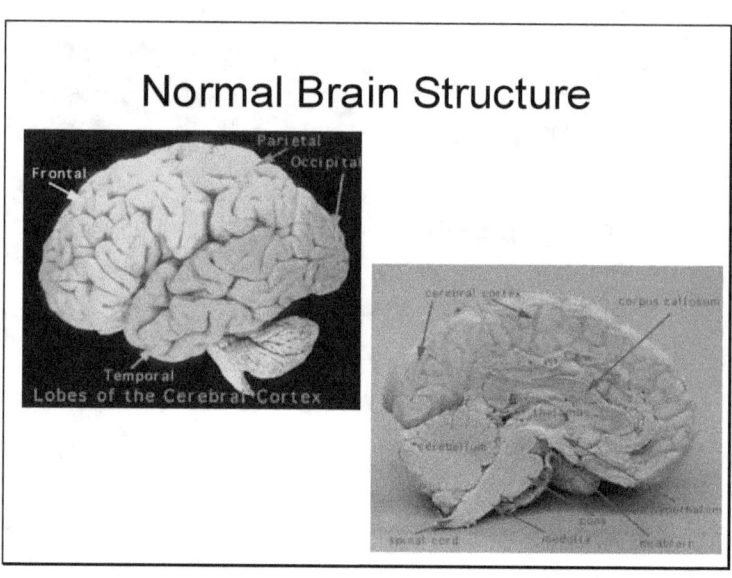

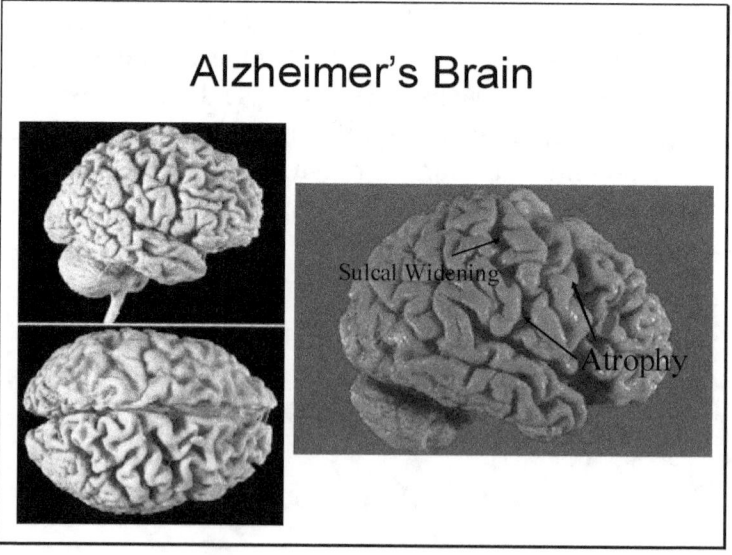

These slides serve as illustrations of how the death of neurons can impact the structure of the brain even on the level of its gross anatomy.

These brains are notable for sulcal the spaces between the gyri
widening....really seen throughout the cortex in the brains on the
left, and seen in the frontal regions of the brain on the right.

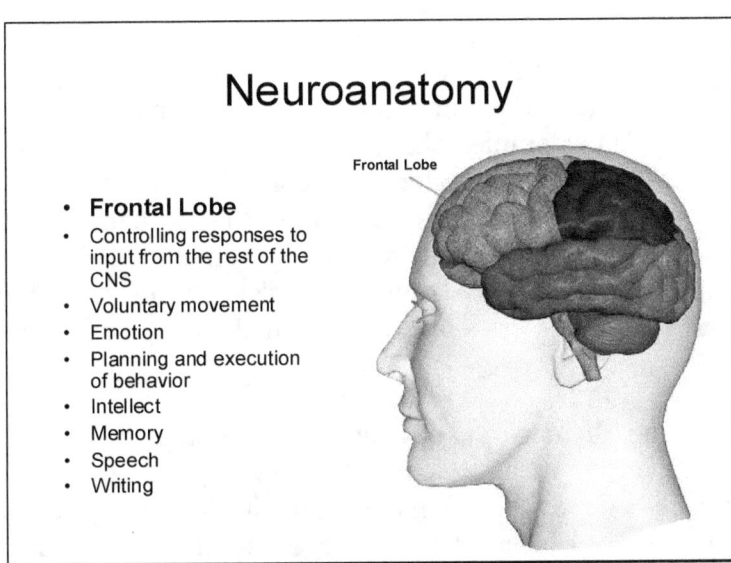

Frontal Lobe is associated with reasoning, planning, parts of
speech, movement, emotions, and problem solving.

Source: (Brain Structures and their Functions)

The frontal lobes are considered the emotional control center and
home to the personality. There is no other part of the brain where
lesions can cause such a wide variety of symptoms (Kolb &
Wishaw, 1990). The frontal lobes are involved in motor function,
problem solving, spontaneity, memory, language, initiation,
judgment, impulse control, and social and sexual behavior. The
frontal lobes are extremely vulnerable to injury due to their
location at the front of the cranium, proximity to the sphenoid wing
and their large size. MRI studies have shown that the frontal area
is the most common region of injury following mild to moderate
traumatic brain injury (Levin et. al., 1987).

There are important asymmetrical differences in the frontal lobes.
The left frontal lobe is involved in controlling language related

movement, whereas the right frontal lobe plays a role in non-verbal abilities. Some researchers emphasize this rule is not absolute and that with many people, both lobes are involved in nearly all behavior.

Disturbance of motor function is typically characterized by loss of fine movements and strength of the arms, hands and fingers (Kuypers, 1981). Complex chains of motor movement also seem to be controlled by the frontal lobes (Leonard et. al., 1988). Patients with frontal lobe damage exhibit little spontaneous facial expression, which points to the role of the frontal lobes in facial expression (Kolb & Milner, 1981). Broca's Aphasia, or difficulty in speaking, has been associated with frontal damage by Brown (1972).

An interesting phenomenon of frontal lobe damage is the insignificant effect it can have on traditional IQ testing. Researchers believe this may have to do with IQ tests typically assessing *convergent* rather than *divergent* thinking. Frontal lobe damage seems to have an impact on divergent thinking, or flexibility and problem solving ability. There is also evidence showing lingering interference with attention and memory even after good recovery from a TBI (Stuss et. al., 1985).

Another area often associated with frontal damage is that of "behavioral spontaneity." Kolb & Milner (1981) found individuals with frontal damage displayed fewer spontaneous facial movements, spoke fewer words (left frontal lesions) or excessively (right frontal lesions).

One of the most common characteristics of frontal lobe damage is difficulty in interpreting feedback from the environment. Perseverating on a response (Milner, 1964), risk taking, and non-compliance with rules (Miller, 1985), and impaired associated learning (using external cues to help guide behavior) (Drewe, 1975) are a few examples of this type of deficit.

The frontal lobes are also thought to play a part in spatial orientation, including the body's orientation in space (Semmes et. al., 1963).

One of the most common effects of frontal damage can be a dramatic change in social behavior. A person's personality can undergo significant changes after an injury to the frontal lobes, especially when both lobes are involved. There are some differences in the left versus right frontal lobes in this area. Left frontal damage usually manifests as pseudodepression and right frontal damage as pseudopsychopathic (Blumer and Benson, 1975).

Sexual behavior can also be affected by frontal lesions. Orbital frontal damage can introduce abnormal sexual behavior, while dorolateral lesions may reduce sexual interest (Walker and Blummer, 1975).

Some common tests for frontal lobe function are: Wisconsin Card Sorting (response inhibition); Finger Tapping (motor skills); Token Test (language skills).

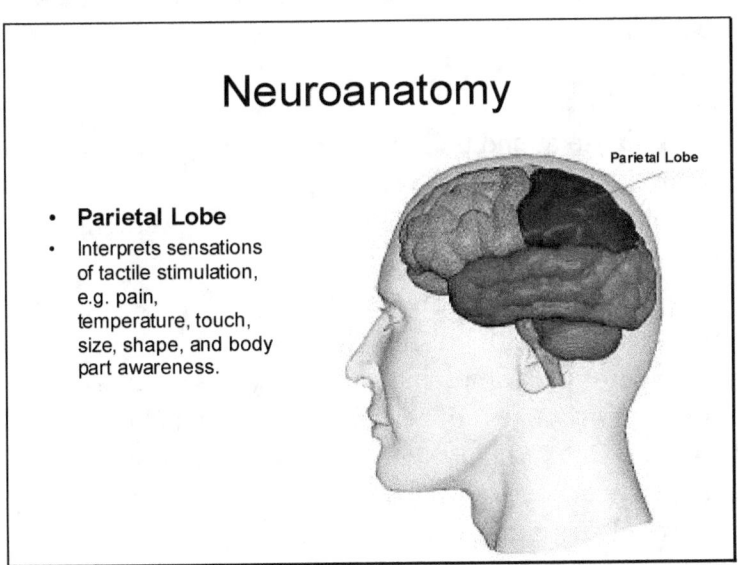

Parietal Lobe is associated with movement, orientation, recognition, perception of stimuli
Sources: (Parietal lobe)

Parietal Lobes
The parietal lobes can be divided into two functional regions. One involves sensation and perception and the other is concerned with integrating sensory input, primarily with the visual system. The first function integrates sensory information to form a single perception (cognition). The second function constructs a spatial coordinate system to represent the world. Individuals with damage to the parietal lobes often show striking deficits, such as abnormalities in body image and spatial relations (Kandel, Schwartz & Jessel, 1991).

Functions:
- Location for visual attention.
- Location for touch perception.
- Goal directed voluntary movements.
- Manipulation of objects.
- Integration of different senses that allows for understanding a single concept.

Observed Problems:
- Inability to attend to more than one object at a time.
- Inability to name an object (Anomia).
- Inability to locate the words for writing (Agraphia).
- Problems with reading (Alexia).
- Difficulty with drawing objects.
- Difficulty in distinguishing left from right.
- Difficulty with doing mathematics (Dyscalculia).
- Lack of awareness of certain body parts and/or surrounding space (Apraxia) that leads to difficulties in self-care.
- Inability to focus visual attention.
- Difficulties with eye and hand coordination.

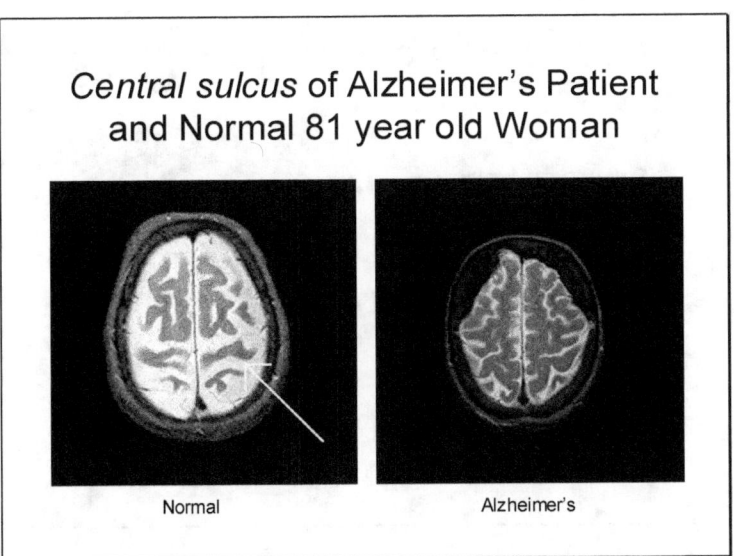

Central sulcus of Alzheimer's Patient
and Normal 81 year old Woman

Normal   Alzheimer's

Source: (Central Sulcus)

The central sulcus is a deep groove (or furrow) in the brain that
separates the frontal and parietal lobes of the cerebrum. The
central sulcus has a 'map' of the human body on each side that
corresponds to the other side. So when the sensory part is
stimulated, its associated motor part is right across the sulcus. The
model of the human body in relation to how many nerves are
associated with each body part is called a homonculus and can be
seen one in one of the pictures above.

Source: (Alzheimer's Disease)
This brain displays many of the commonest features of the disease:
brain shrinkage, or atrophy, and loss of function, as indicated by
hypoperfusion. First, look at the prominent sulci, especially the
central sulcus. Some reduction in brain volume is a part of normal
aging, but compare this brain with the normal central sulcus, from
a normal 81 year old woman. The abnormal shrinkage seen in this
case, while not a finding specific to Alzheimer's disease, is severe
and seems to affect some regions more than others.

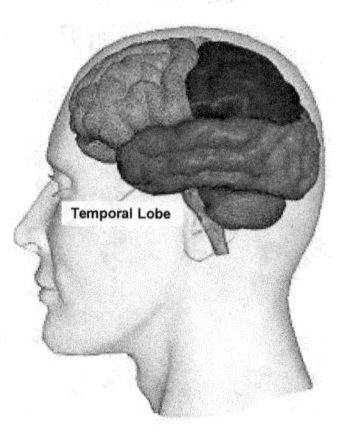

Neuroanatomy

- **Temporal Lobe**
  - Understanding sounds
  - Understanding speech
  - Emotion
  - Memory

Temporal Lobe

Source: (Centre for Neuro Skills)

Temporal Lobe is associated with perception and recognition of auditory stimuli, memory, and speech.

Temporal Lobes
Kolb & Wishaw (1990) have identified eight principle symptoms of temporal lobe damage: 1) disturbance of auditory sensation and perception, 2) disturbance of selective attention of auditory and visual input, 3) disorders of visual perception, 4) impaired organization and categorization of verbal material, 5) disturbance of language comprehension, 6) impaired long-term memory, 7) altered personality and affective behavior, and 8) altered sexual behavior.

Functions:
- Hearing ability.
- Memory acquisition.
- Some visual perceptions.
- Categorization of objects.

Observed Problems:
- Difficulty in recognizing faces (Prosopagnosia).
- Difficulty in understanding spoken words (Wernicke's Aphasia).
- Disturbance with selective attention to what we see and hear.
- Difficulty with identification of, and verbalization about objects.
- Short-term memory loss.
- Interference with long-term memory
- Increased or decreased interest in sexual behavior.
- Inability to categorize objects (Categorization).
- Right lobe damage can cause persistent talking.
- Increased aggressive behavior.

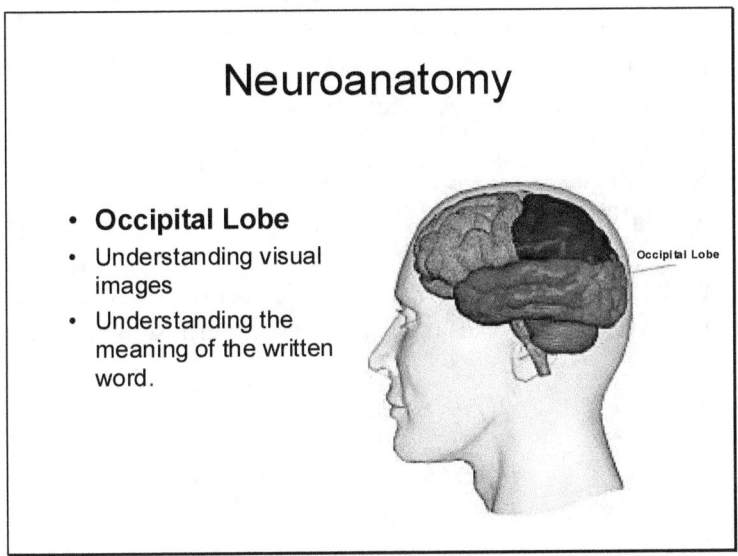

Neuroanatomy

- **Occipital Lobe**
- Understanding visual images
- Understanding the meaning of the written word.

Source: (Centre for Neuro Skills)

Occipital Lobe is associated with visual processing.

Occipital Lobes
The occipital lobes are the center of visual perception system. They are not particularly vulnerable to injury because of their location at the back of the brain, although any significant trauma to

the brain could produce subtle changes to the visual-perceptual system, such as visual field defects and scotomas.

Functions:
- Vision.

Observed Problems:
- Defects in vision (Visual Field Cuts).
- Difficulty with locating objects in environment.
- Difficulty with identifying colors (Color Agnosia).
- Production of hallucinations.
- Visual illusions - inaccurately seeing objects.
- Word blindness - inability to recognize words.
- Difficulty in recognizing drawn objects.
- Inability to recognize the movement of an object (Movement Agnosia).
- Difficulties with reading and writing.
- Consolidation of New Memories.
- Emotions.
- Navigation.
- Spatial Orientation.

The hippocampus is a horseshoe shaped sheet of neurons located within the temporal lobes and adjacent to the amygdala.

Neuroanatomy

- **Hippocampus**
- Plays crucial role in both encoding and retrieval of information
- Damage to hippocampus produces *global retrograde amnesia*, inability to retain newly learned information

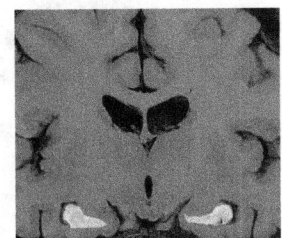

Source: (Med.Sci 532)

Hippocampus (hippo camp' us)
 is tucked out of sight on the medial side of the temporal lobe. It is important for converting short term memory to more permanent memory, and for recalling spatial relationships in the world. It is also part of the limbic lobe. It received its name because its shape resembles that of a 'seahorse'.

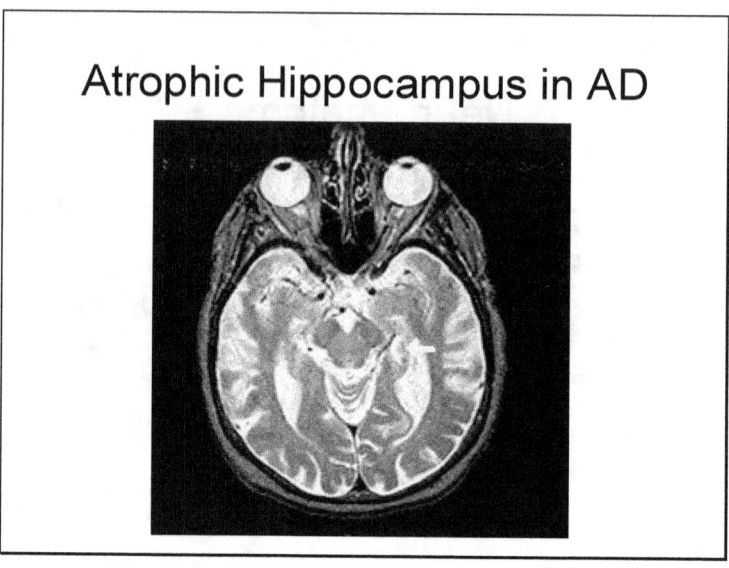

Atrophic Hippocampus in AD

An early marker for AD is atrophy, a wasting or decrease in size.

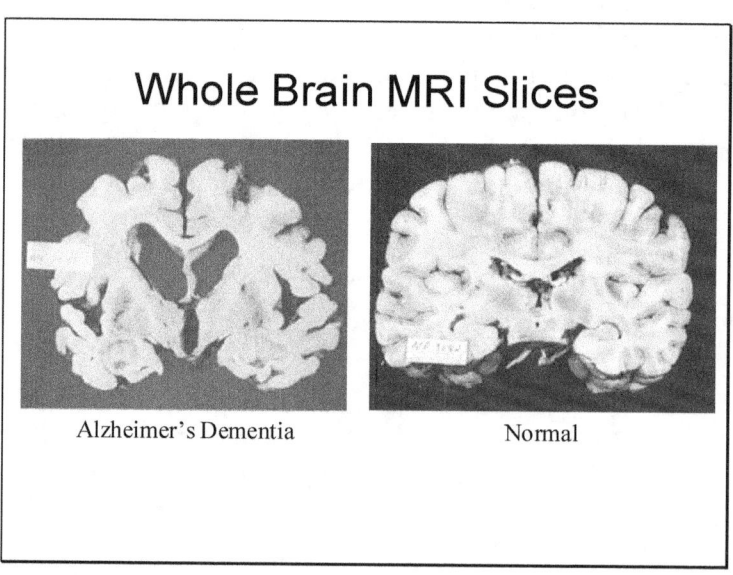

Whole Brain MRI Slices

Alzheimer's Dementia   Normal

Source: (About.com)
Alzheimer's disease is a progressive process of brain degeneration.
Deterioration in brain function due to Alzheimer's usually
progresses as:

- Learning and memory difficulties.
- Planning and judgment difficulties.
- Speech problems.
- Orientation problems.
- Major impact on Activities of Daily Life (ADLs).
- Bodily functions.

Degeneration of Basal Ganglia

- Huntington's disease
  - Rare: 5 in 100,000
  - Abnormal 'exagerated' movements

- Parkinson's disease
  - Common: 1 in 100 over age 65
  - General slowing of voluntary movements

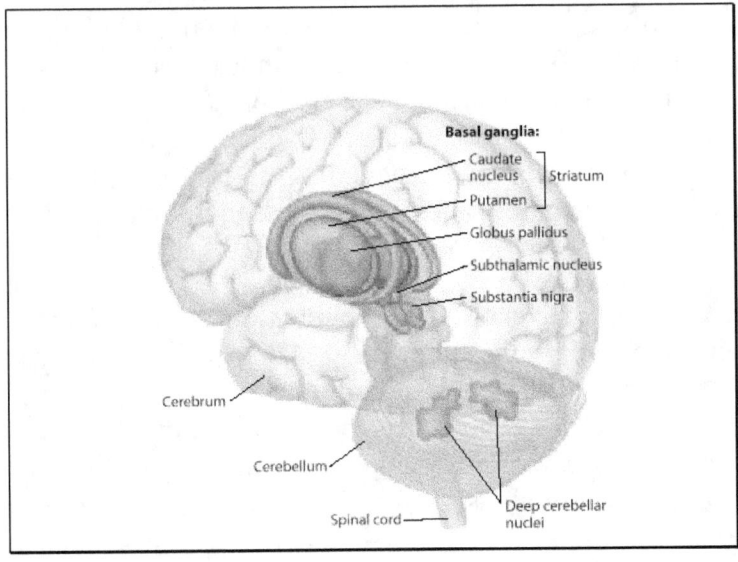

Source: (Wikipedia)
Basal Ganglia: The basal ganglia are a group of large nuclei that partially surround the thalamus. These nuclei are important in the control of movement. The red nucleus and substantia nigra of the midbrain have connections with the basal ganglia:

- Controls Cognition.
- Movement Coordination.
- Voluntary Movement.

The basal ganglia is located deep within the cerebral hemispheres in the telencephalon region of the brain. It consists of the corpus stratium, subthalamic nucleus and the substantia nigra.

Source: (Cleveland Clinic)
Huntington's disease, also called **Huntington's chorea, chorea major**, or **HD**, is a genetic neurological disorder characterized after onset by uncoordinated, jerky body movements and a decline in some mental abilities. These characteristics vary per individual, physical ones less so, but the differing decline in mental abilities can lead to a number of potential behavioral problems. The disorder itself isn't fatal, but as symptoms progress, complications reducing life expectancy increase. Research of HD has increased greatly in the last few decades, but its exact mechanism is unknown, so symptoms are managed individually. Globally, up to 7 people in 100,000 have the disorder, although there are localized regions with a higher incidence. Onset of physical symptoms occurs gradually and can begin at any age, although it is statistically most common in a person's mid-forties (with a 30 year spread). If onset is before age twenty, the condition is classified as juvenile HD.

A physical and/or psychological examination can determine whether initial symptoms are evident. Abnormal movements are often the symptoms that cause initial impetus to seek medical consultation and lead to diagnosis; however, the disease may begin with cognitive or psychiatric symptoms, which are not always recognized except in hindsight, or if they develop further. Pre-symptomatic testing is possible using a blood test which counts the numbers of CAG repeats in each of the HTT alleles, although a positive result is not considered a diagnosis, since it may be obtained decades before onset of symptoms. A negative blood test means that the individual does not carry the expanded copy of the gene. A full pathological diagnosis can only be established by a neurological examination's findings and/or demonstration of cell loss in the areas affected by HD, supported by a cranial CT or MRI scan findings.

A pre-symptomatic test is a life-changing event and a very personal decision. The personal ramifications to an at-risk individual and lack of cure for the disease necessitate several counseling sessions to ensure that they are prepared for either result before it is given. In England, Scotland, Northern Ireland, Australia, Canada and New Zealand, unless a person under eighteen years of age is considered to be Gillick competent, testing is not considered ethical - unless they show significant symptoms, or are sexually active. Many organizations and lay groups strongly endorse these restrictions in their testing protocol.

Embryonic screening is also possible, giving affected or at-risk individuals the option of ensuring their children will not inherit the disease. It is possible for women who would consider abortion of an affected fetus to test an embryo in the womb (prenatal diagnosis). Other techniques, such as preimplantation genetic diagnosis in the setting of in vitro fertilization, can be used to ensure that the newborn is unaffected.

Management
Treatments for cognitive and psychological symptoms include antidepressants and sedatives, and low doses of antipsychotics. There is limited evidence for specific treatments aimed at controlling the chorea and other movement abnormalities, although tetrabenazine has been shown to reduce the severity of the chorea; it was approved in 2008 specifically for this indication.

Nutrition management is an important part of treatment; most people in the later stages of the disease need more calories than average to maintain body weight. Thickening agent can be added to drinks as swallowing becomes more difficult, as thicker fluids are easier and safer to swallow. The option of using a percutaneous endoscopic gastrostomy (i.e., a feeding tube into the stomach) is available when eating becomes too hazardous or uncomfortable. A "stomach PEG" greatly reduces the chances of aspiration of food, which can lead to aspiration pneumonia, and also increases the amount of nutrients and calories that can be ingested, aiding the body's natural defenses.

Although there are relatively few studies of rehabilitation for HD, its general effectiveness when conducted by a team of specialists has been clearly demonstrated in other pathologies such as stroke, or head trauma. As for any patient with neurologic deficits, a multidisciplinary approach is key to limiting and overcoming disability. There is some evidence for the usefulness of physical therapy and speech therapy but more rigorous studies are needed for health authorities to endorse them.

Source: (BNET's Buisness Owners)

Parkinsons' Disease

Overview

Parkinson's disease (PD) was first described in 1817 by Dr. James Parkinson, a British physician, for whom the disease was named. It is a disease that is characterized by four major features:

- Rest tremor of a limb (shaking with the limb at rest).
- Slowness of movement (bradykinesia).
- Rigidity (stiffness, increased resistance to passive movement) of the limbs or trunk.
- Poor balance (postural instability).

When at least two of these symptoms are present, and especially if they are more evident on one side than the other, a diagnosis of PD is made, unless there are atypical features that suggest an alternative diagnosis. Patients may first realize something is wrong when they develop a tremor in a limb; movements are slowed and activities take longer to perform; or they experience stiffness and have balance problems. Initially, symptoms are a variable combination of tremor, bradykinesia, rigidity, and postural instability. Symptoms typically begin on one side of the body and spread over time to the other side.

Changes occur in facial expression, so that there is a certain facial fixity (blank expression showing little emotion) or a staring appearance (due to reduced frequency of eye blinking). Complaints of a frozen shoulder or foot drag on the affected side are not uncommon. As symptoms come on gradually, older patients may attribute these changes to aging. The tremor is thought to be "shakiness," bradykinesia is regarded as normal "slowing down," and stiffness is attributed to arthritis. The stooped posture, common to PD, may be attributed to age or osteoporosis. Both younger and older patients may experience initial symptoms for a year or more before seeking medical evaluation.

Parkinson's disease affects 1 in 100 people over the age of 60, with the average age of onset being 60 years. It can also affect younger people. Young-onset Parkinson's disease (onset at age 40 or younger) is estimated to occur in 5 – 10% of patients with PD.

Disease Progression
After Alzheimer's disease, Parkinson's disease is the most common neurodegenerative disease.

It is a chronic, progressive disease that results when nerve cells in a part of the midbrain, called the substantia nigra, die, or are impaired. These nerve cells produce dopamine, an important chemical messenger that transmits signals from the substantia nigra to another part of the brain called the corpus striatum. These signals allow for coordinated movement. When the dopamine-secreting cells in the substantia nigra die, the other movement control centers in the brain become unregulated. These disturbances in the control centers of the brain cause the symptoms of PD. When 80% of the dopamine-producing cells in the substantia nigra are depleted, symptoms of PD develop.

Initially the symptoms are mild, usually on one side of the body, and may not require medical treatment. Rest tremor is a major characteristic of PD, and the most common presenting symptom, but some patients never develop it. Tremor may be the least disabling symptom, but is often the most embarrassing to the patient. Patients may keep their affected hand in their pocket, behind their back, or hold something to control the tremor, which may be more psychologically distressing than any physical limitation that it imposes.

Over time, initial symptoms become worse. A mild tremor becomes more bothersome and more noticeable. Difficulties may develop with cutting food or handling utensils with the affected limb. Bradykinesia (slowness in movement) becomes a significant problem and the most disabling symptom. Slowness may interfere with daily routines; getting dressed, shaving, or showering may take much of the day. Mobility is impaired and difficulty develops in getting into or out of a chair or a car, or turning over in bed. Walking is slower and there is a stooped posture, with the head and shoulders hanging forward. The voice becomes soft and monotonous. A disturbance of balance may lead to falls. Handwriting becomes small ("micrographia") and illegible. Automatic movements, such as arm swing when walking, are reduced.

Symptoms may originally be restricted to one limb, but will typically spread over time to the other limb on the same side. They eventually progress to the other side of the body. Generally this progression is gradual, but the rate of progression varies in different patients. As symptoms progress, it is important for patients to talk with their physicians so that optimal treatment can be established. The goal of treatment is not to abolish symptoms, but rather to help the patient manage their symptoms, function independently, and make the appropriate adjustments to a chronic illness. The illness will not go away, but management of its symptoms can be successful in reducing disability or other handicap.

Patients are aware of the progressive nature of the illness and this may become a source of much anxiety. It is not uncommon for patients to over-monitor themselves and their symptoms, compare themselves to other Parkinson's disease patients whom they may meet (length of diagnosis, level of symptoms, etc.), and avoid situations such as support groups, where they may see patients who are worse off than they are. Concern about the progression of the disease and the ability to continue working is frequently voiced.

It is not possible to predict with any confidence the likely course of the disease in an individual patient. The rate of progression and resulting level of disability vary in different patients. Some guide to the likely outcome in individual patients is provided by the course of the illness since diagnosis, but this is no more than suggestive.

When the disorder is such that normal activities of daily living are impaired, at least to some extent, symptomatic treatment is begun.

Summary

- The most complex mass in the universe

- Functional Location
  - Relevant
  - Differ in some naturally
  - Can change with injury

- Functional Plasticity

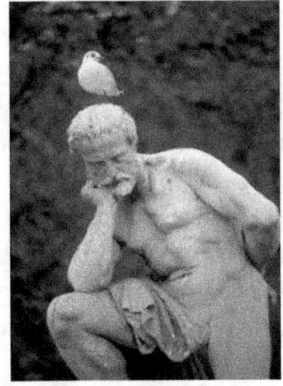

There is no known structure more complex than the three pounds of material atop the shoulders in the human skull. With over 100 billion neurons, each contacting to thousands of others its ability to remember, anticipate, plan, organize, recognize, etc. are unsurpassed by any super computer.

Functional localization is often misunderstood. The preceding pages discussed areas of the brain primarily responsible for certain functions. However, "primarily" is the key phrase, the brain is a singular unit, operating with a remarkable cooperation from all parts. For example, memory is involved in processing sound, sight, touch and even taste and smell. To say the temporal lobe processes language is only part of the story. In fact, the temporal lobe processes the structure of language (i.e., the words). It plays a very important role in constructing sentences and maintaining coherent expression and temporal flow of information. However, other parts of the brain interprets the emotion of the words used; another part reads the gestures and other non-verbal parts of the message; and still others brings to awareness the context in which the message is delivered. This is only a small part of what goes on during every conversation in the health brain. Most people have all misinterpreted just one aspect of a message and totally misunderstood the message. One of the most hideous aspects of dementia is the removal of some, not all, of these abilities. The client begins to misunderstand verbal communication. Not due to a lack of understanding the words, but from a misreading of one or more of the other parts of the message (i.e., gestures, tone, volume, cadence, inflections, etc.).

The healthy brain is fully engaged. At no time do humans use just 10% of their brains. Humans recognize less than their full cognitive potential, but this results in fewer neuron connections not in parts of the brain being unused. Learning, experiencing, and being active create new neuron connections. Through these connections relationships are formed between newly learned information and previously learned information; new experiences with prior ones; new activities with prior ones. This is essentially how the brain learns – by relating newly learned knowledge and/or experiences with prior knowledge and experiences. The brain is associative so the more one knows the easier it is to associate new knowledge.

Another important point about brain localization is its plasticity – its ability to move the primary processing area to another part of the brain when the primary area is damaged. This process may take years of retraining. Medical journals often reference remarkable recoveries after brain injuries as proof of this plasticity. Continuous re-learning and optimism is the best practice for clients with brain injuries. There is still much to learn about the function of the brain. Every day brings new understanding which leads to new interventions. As care givers for those with dementia an occasional review of recent research and continuing education is essential to meeting the client's needs.

Works Cited

About.com. (n.d.). *How The Brain Changes During Alzheimer's Diseas*. Retrieved Oct 2010, from http://alzheimers.about.com/od/caregivers/ig/Brain-Changes-in-Alzheimer-s/

Azzheimer's Disease. (n.d.). Retrieved Apr 2009, from Harvard Medical: http://www.med.harvard.edu/AANLIB/cases/case3/mr1/040.html

BNET's Buisness Owners. (n.d.). *Deep Brain Stimulation for Advanced Parkinson's Disease*. Retrieved Oct 2010, from The CBS Interactive Business Network: http://findarticles.com/p/articles/mi_m0FSL/is_3_72/ai_65539091/

Brain Structures and their Functions. (n.d.). Retrieved Oct 2010, from Serendip: http://serendip.brynmawr.edu/bb/kinser/Structure1.html

Central Sulcus. (n.d.). Retrieved Oct 2010, from KeyWen: http://keywen.com/en/CENTRAL_SULCUS

Centre for Neuro Skills. (n.d.). *Occipital Lobes*. Retrieved Oct 2010, from http://www.neuroskills.com/tbi/boccipit.shtml

Cleveland Clinic. (n.d.). *Huntington's Disease*. Retrieved Sept 2010, from http://my.clevelandclinic.org/disorders/huntingtons_disease/hic_huntingtons_disease.aspx

DementiaGuide. (n.d.). *Dementia vs. Alzheimer's*. Retrieved Oct 2010, from Dementia Guide: http://www.dementiaguide.com/community/dementia-articles/Dementia_vs_Alzheimer's:_clearing_the_confusion

Med.Sci 532. (n.d.). *Hippocampus*. Retrieved 2010 Oct, from http://www.sci.uidaho.edu/med532/hippocam.htm

Parietal lobe. (n.d.). Retrieved Oct 2010, from Wikipedia: http://en.wikipedia.org/wiki/Parietal_lobe

Paul, K. L. (2005). *The Aging Population and the Relevance of Vascular Dementia*. Retrieved Oct 2010, from Google Books: http://books.google.com/books?id=I-wEfVhRKEIC&pg=PA4&lpg=PA4&dq=By+2030,+there+are+expected+to+be+70+million++dementia&source=bl&

ots=946er0XIv7&sig=_X1qeq4Lqjt6wTyyIp4Cc37dkQQ&
hl=en&ei=Oe7VTLDHHIr0swPL_fCMCw&sa=X&oi=boo
k_result&ct=result&resnum=1&ved=0CBc

Pekker, M. (n.d.). *Diagnostic criteria of Dementia of the Alzheimer's Type*. Retrieved Oct 2010, from Alzheimer's disease: Causes, Symptoms, Treatment: http://alzheimers-review.blogspot.com/2010/09/diagnostic-criteria-of-dementia-of.html

Skills, C. f. (n.d.). *Temporal Lobes*. Retrieved Oct 2010, from TBI Resource Guide: http://www.neuroskills.com/tbi/btemporl.shtml

Wikipedia. (n.d.). *Basal Ganglia*. Retrieved Oct 2010, from http://en.wikipedia.org/wiki/Basal_ganglia

Chapter 2 – Dementia Diagnosis

Differential Diagnosis: Top Ten
(commonly used mnemonic device: AVDEMENTIA)

1. Alzheimer Disease
2. Vascular Disease
3. Drugs, Depression, Delirium
4. Ethanol
5. Medical / Metabolic Systems
6. Endocrine (thyroid, diabetes), Ears, Eyes, Environment
7. Neurologic (other primary degenerations, etc.)
8. Tumor, Toxin, Trauma
9. Infection, Idiopathic, Immunologic
10. Amnesia, Autoimmune, Apnea, AAMI

Diagnosis of Dementia

* Memory Impairment AND one of the following:

   -Aphasia, Apraxia, Agnosia, or Impaired Executive Functioning

* Deficits cause significant impairment in social or occupational functions

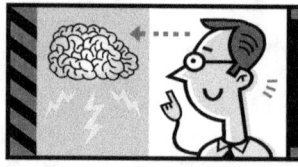

The diagnosis of dementia rests upon the finding of memory impairment and at least one other "cognitive" deficit. By DSM-IV, criteria, these include aphasia, apraxia, agnosia or impaired executive functioning. Aphasia in these patients can refer to word finding deficits or more severe problems with language. Apraxia is an inability to perform some type of motor function in the absence of an actual motor deficit. An example of this may be the inability to use a common household item correctly such as a vacuum cleaner, or an inability to use a doorknob. Agnosia means an inability to recognize things in the outside world for example, faces of people or objects.

Executive functioning refers to the individual's ability to plan, imagine, and think in an abstract way. To be listed as a disorder of any kind, these deficits must be of sufficient severity to cause a major decrease in level of functioning.

Aphasia

- Characterized initially by a fluent aphasia
  - Initiate and maintain a conversation
  - Impaired comprehension
  - Intact grammar and syntax however speech is vague with paraphasias, circumlocutions, tangential and nonspecific phrases ("the thing")
  - Later language can be severely impaired with mutism, echolalia

Source: (The National Aphasia Association)
Aphasia is an acquired communication disorder that impairs a person's ability to process language, but does not affect intelligence. Aphasia impairs the ability to speak and understand others, and most people with aphasia experience difficulty reading and writing.

What causes aphasia?
The most common cause of aphasia is stroke (about 25-40% of

stroke survivors acquire aphasia). It can also result from head injury, brain tumor or other neurological causes.

How common is aphasia?
Aphasia affects about one million Americans -or 1 in 250 people- and is more common than Parkinson's Disease, cerebral palsy or muscular dystrophy. More than 100,000 Americans acquire the disorder each year. However, most people have never heard of it.

Who acquires aphasia?
While aphasia is most common among older people, it can occur in people of all ages, races, nationalities, and gender.

Can a Person Have Aphasia Without Having a Physical Disability?
Yes, but many people with aphasia also have weakness or paralysis of their right leg and right arm. When a person acquires aphasia it is usually due to damage on the left side of the brain, which controls movements on the right side of the body.

Can People Who Have Aphasia Return to Their Jobs?
Sometimes. Since most jobs require speech and language skills, aphasia can make some types of work difficult. Individuals with mild or even moderate aphasia are sometimes able to work, but they may have to change jobs. Some resources for aphasics looking for work are as follows:

*National Organization on Disability (NOD), www.nod.org, (202) 293-5960. *Lists organizations recruiting and/or assisting people with disabilities in securing jobs.*

*Job Accommodation Network, www.jan.wvu.edu, (800) 526-7234. *Help to find employment and links to organization recruiting/assisting with disabilities in finding a job. Information on small business/self-employment.*

*DisabliityInfo.gov, www.disabilityinfo.gov. *Government disability website. Has a handbook on job-seeking skills for people with disabilities.*

*Equal Employment Opportunity Commission (EEOC), www.eeoc.gov, (800) 669-4000. *ADA information and instructions on how to file complaints. Free booklets on regulations and guidelines for the ADA.*

How long does it take to recover from Aphasia?
If the symptoms of aphasia last longer than two or three months after a stroke, a complete recovery is unlikely. However, it is important to note that some people continue to improve over a period of years and even decades. Improvement is a slow process that usually involves both helping the individual and family understand the nature of aphasia and learning compensatory strategies for communicating.

Does Aphasia affect a person's intelligence?
No. A person with aphasia may have difficulty retrieving words and names, but the person's intelligence is basically intact. Aphasia is not like Alzheimer's disease; for people with aphasia it is the ability to access ideas and thoughts through language - not the ideas and thoughts themselves- that is disrupted. But because people with aphasia have difficulty communicating, others often mistakenly assume they are mentally ill or have mental retardation.

Are all cases of Aphasia alike?
No. There are many types of aphasia. Some people have difficulty speaking while others may struggle to follow a conversation. In some people, aphasia is fairly mild and one may not notice it right away. In other cases, it can be very severe, affecting speaking, writing, reading, and listening. While specific symptoms can vary greatly, what all people with aphasia have in common are difficulties in communicating.

Communicating with people who have Aphasia: some "do's & don'ts"
Aphasia is a communication impairment usually acquired as a result of a stroke or other brain injury. It affects both the ability to express oneself through speech, gesture, and writing, and to understand the speech, gesture, and writing of others. Aphasia

thus changes the way in which we communicate with those people most important to us: family, friends, and co-workers. The impact of aphasia on relationships may be profound, or only slight. No two people with aphasia are alike with respect to severity, former speech and language skills, or personality. But in all cases it is essential for the person to communicate as successfully as possible from the very beginning of the recovery process. Here are some suggestions to help communicate with a person with aphasia:

- Make sure to have the person's attention before communicating.
- During conversation, minimize or eliminate background noise (such as television, radio, and other people) as much as possible.
- Keep communication simple but adult. Simplify sentence structure and reduce the rate of speech. One does not need to speak louder than normal but do emphasize key words. Do not talk down to the person with aphasia.
- Encourage and use other modes of communication (writing, drawing, yes/no responses, choices, gestures, eye contact, facial expressions) in addition to speech.
- Give them time to talk and let them have a reasonable amount of time to respond. Avoid speaking for the person with aphasia except when necessary and ask permission before doing so.
- Praise all attempts to speak; make speaking a pleasant experience and provide stimulating conversation. Downplay errors and avoid frequent criticisms/corrections. Avoid insisting that each word be produced perfectly.
- Augment speech with gesture and visual aids whenever possible. Repeat a statement when necessary.
- Encourage them to be as independent as possible. Avoid being overprotective.
- Whenever possible continue normal activities (such as dinner with family, company, going out). Do not shield people with aphasia from family or friends or ignore them in a group conversation. Rather, try to involve them in family decision-making as much as possible. Keep them

informed of events but avoid burdening them with day to day details.

Apraxia

- Inability to carry out motor activities despite intact motor function
  - Contributes to loss of Activities of Daily Living (ADLs)

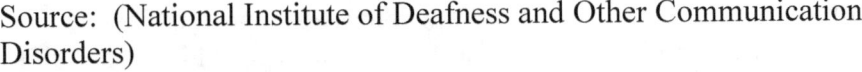

Source: (National Institute of Deafness and Other Communication Disorders)

What is apraxia of speech?
Apraxia of speech, also known as verbal apraxia or dyspraxia, is a speech disorder in which a person has trouble saying what he or she wants to say correctly and consistently. It is not due to weakness or paralysis of the speech muscles (the muscles of the face, tongue, and lips). The severity of apraxia of speech can range from mild to severe.

What are the types and causes of apraxia?
There are two main types of speech apraxia: acquired apraxia of speech and developmental apraxia of speech. Acquired apraxia of speech can affect a person at any age, although it most typically occurs in adults. It is caused by damage to the parts of the brain that are involved in speaking, and involves the loss or impairment of existing speech abilities. The disorder may result from a stroke, head injury, tumor, or other illness affecting the brain. Acquired apraxia of speech may occur together with muscle weakness

affecting speech production (dysarthria) or language difficulties caused by damage to the nervous system (aphasia).

Developmental Apraxia of Speech (DAS) occurs in children and is present from birth. It appears to affect more boys than girls. This speech disorder goes by several other names, including developmental verbal apraxia, developmental verbal dyspraxia, articulatory apraxia, and childhood apraxia of speech. DAS is different from what is known as a developmental delay of speech, in which a child follows the "typical" path of speech development but does so more slowly than normal.

The cause or causes of DAS are not yet known. Some scientists believe that DAS is a disorder related to a child's overall language development. Others believe it is a neurological disorder that affects the brain's ability to send the proper signals to move the muscles involved in speech. However, brain imaging and other studies have not found evidence of specific brain lesions or differences in brain structure in children with DAS. Children with DAS often have family members who have a history of communication disorders or learning disabilities. This observation and recent research findings suggest that genetic factors may play a role in the disorder.

What are the symptoms?
People with either form of apraxia of speech may have a number of different speech characteristics, or symptoms. One of the most notable symptoms is difficulty putting sounds and syllables together in the correct order to form words. Longer or more complex words are usually harder to say than shorter or simpler words. People with apraxia of speech also tend to make inconsistent mistakes when speaking. For example, they may say a difficult word correctly but then have trouble repeating it, or they may be able to say a particular sound one day and have trouble with the same sound the next day. People with apraxia of speech often appear to be groping for the right sound or word, and may try saying a word several times before they say it correctly.

Another common characteristic of apraxia of speech is the incorrect use of "prosody" -- that is, the varying rhythms, stresses, and inflections of speech that are used to help express meaning.

Children with developmental apraxia of speech generally can understand language much better than they are able to use language to express themselves. Some children with the disorder may also have other problems. These can include other speech problems, such as dysarthria; language problems such as poor vocabulary, incorrect grammar, and difficulty in clearly organizing spoken information; problems with reading, writing, spelling, or math; coordination or "motor-skill" problems; and chewing and swallowing difficulties.

The severity of both acquired and developmental apraxia of speech varies from person to person. Apraxia can be so mild that a person has trouble with very few speech sounds or only has occasional problems pronouncing words with many syllables. In the most severe cases, a person may not be able to communicate effectively with speech, and may need the help of alternative or additional communication methods.

How is it diagnosed?
Professionals known as speech-language pathologists play a key role in diagnosing and treating apraxia of speech. There is no single factor or test that can be used to diagnose apraxia. In addition, speech-language experts do not agree about which specific symptoms are part of developmental apraxia. The person making the diagnosis generally looks for the presence of some, or many, of a group of symptoms, including those described above. Ruling out other contributing factors, such as muscle weakness or language-comprehension problems, can also help with the diagnosis.

To diagnose developmental apraxia of speech, parents and professionals may need to observe a child's speech over a period of time. In formal testing for both acquired and developmental apraxia, the speech-language pathologist may ask the person to perform speech tasks such as repeating a particular word several times or repeating a list of words of increasing length (for example, *love, loving, lovingly*). For acquired apraxia of speech, a speech-language pathologist may also examine a person's ability to converse, read, write, and perform non-speech movements. Brain-imaging tests such as magnetic resonance imaging (MRI) may also be used to help distinguish acquired apraxia of speech from other communication disorders in people who have experienced brain damage.

How is it treated?
In some cases, people with acquired apraxia of speech recover some or all of their speech abilities on their own. This is called spontaneous recovery. Children with developmental apraxia of speech will not outgrow the problem on their own. Speech-language therapy is often helpful for these children and for people with acquired apraxia who do not spontaneously recover all of their speech abilities.

Speech-language pathologists use different approaches to treat apraxia of speech, and no single approach has been proven to be the most effective. Therapy is tailored to the individual and is designed to treat other speech or language problems that may occur together with apraxia. Each person responds differently to therapy, and some people will make more progress than others. People with apraxia of speech usually need frequent and intensive one-on-one therapy. Support and encouragement from family members and friends are also important.

In severe cases, people with acquired or developmental apraxia of speech may need to use other ways to express themselves. These might include formal or informal sign language, a language notebook with pictures or written words that the person can show to other people, or an electronic communication device such as a portable computer that writes and produces speech.

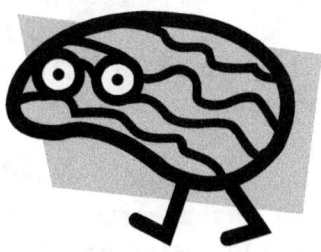

Agnosia

- Inability to recognize or identify objects despite intact sensory function
  - Typically occurs later in course of illness
  - Can be visual or tactile

Source: (Merck)
Agnosia is inability to identify an object using one or more of the senses. Diagnosis is clinical, often including neuropsychological testing, with brain imaging (e.g., CT, MRI) to identify the cause. Prognosis depends on the nature and extent of damage and client age. There is no specific treatment, but occupational therapy may help patients compensate.

Agnosias are uncommon. They result from damage to (e.g., by infarct, tumor, trauma) or degeneration of areas of the brain that integrate perception, memory, and identification.

Discrete brain lesions can cause different forms of agnosia, which may involve any sense. Typically, only one sense is affected. Examples are hearing (auditory agnosia, the inability to identify objects through sound such as a ringing telephone), taste (gustatory agnosia), smell (olfactory agnosia), touch (tactile agnosia), and sight (visual agnosia).

Other forms of agnosia involve very specific and complex processes within one sense. For example, prosopagnosia is inability to identify well-known faces, including those of close friends, or to otherwise distinguish individual objects among a class of objects, despite the ability to identify generic facial features and objects.

Anosognosia often accompanies damage to the right, non-dominant parietal lobe. Patients deny their deficit, insisting that nothing is wrong even when one side of their body is completely paralyzed. When shown the paralyzed body part, patients may deny that it is theirs. In an often related phenomenon, patients ignore the paralyzed or desensitized body parts (hemi-inattention) or the space around them (hemineglect). Hemineglect most often involves the left side of the body.

Occipito-temporal lesions may cause an inability to recognize familiar places (environmental agnosia), visual disturbances (visual agnosia), or color blindness (achromatopsia). Right-sided temporal lesions may cause an inability to interpret sounds (auditory agnosia) or impaired music perception (amusia).

Diagnosis
- At bedside, patients are asked to identify common objects through sight, touch, or another sense. If hemineglect is suspected, patients are asked to identify the paralyzed parts of their body or objects in their hemivisual fields. Physical examination is done to detect primary deficits in individual senses or communication that may interfere with testing for agnosias. For example, if light touch is defective, patients may not sense an object even when cortical function is intact. Also, aphasias may interfere with client's expression. Neuropsychological testing may help identify more subtle agnosias.
- Brain imaging (e.g., CT or MRI with or without angiographic protocols) is required to characterize a central lesion (e.g., infarct, hemorrhage, and mass) and to check for atrophy suggesting a degenerative disorder.

Prognosis
Recovery may be influenced by size and location of lesions, degree of impairment, and client age. Most recovery occurs within the first 3 months but may continue to a variable degree up to a year.

Treatment

There is no specific treatment. Rehabilitation with speech or occupational therapists can help patients learn to compensate for their deficits.

Impaired Executive Function

- Difficulty with planning, initiating, sequencing, monitoring, or stopping complex behaviors.
  - Occurs early to mid-stage
  - Contributes to loss of instrumental of ADLs such as shopping, meal preparation, driving, and managing finances

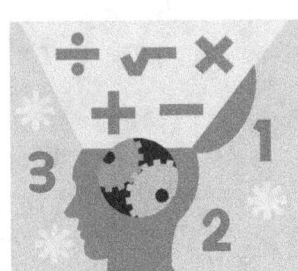

Source: (Encyclopedia of Mental Disorders)

Definition

The term executive function describes a set of cognitive abilities that control and regulate other abilities and behaviors. Executive functions are necessary for goal-directed behavior. They include the ability to initiate and stop actions, to monitor and change behavior as needed, and to plan future behavior when faced with novel tasks and situations. Executive functions allow us to anticipate outcomes and adapt to changing situations. The ability to form concepts and think abstractly is often considered components of executive function.

Description

As the name implies, executive functions are high-level abilities that influence more basic abilities like attention, memory, and motor skills. For this reason, they can be difficult to assess directly. Many of the tests used to measure other abilities, particularly those that look at more complex aspects of these abilities, can be used to evaluate executive functions. For example, a person with executive function deficits may perform well on tests of basic attention, such as those that simply ask the individual to look at a computer screen and respond when a particular shape appears, but have trouble with tasks that require divided or alternating attention, such as giving a different response depending on the stimulus presented. Verbal fluency tests that ask people to say a number of words in a certain period of time can also reveal problems with executive function. One commonly used test asks individuals to name as many animals or as many words beginning with a particular letter as they can in one minute.

A person with executive function deficits may find the animal naming task simple, but struggle to name words beginning with a particular letter, since this task requires people to organize concepts in a novel way. Executive functions also influence memory abilities by allowing people to employ strategies that can help them remember information. Other tests are designed to assess cognitive function more directly. Such tests may present a fairly simple task but without instructions on how to complete it. Executive functions allow most people to figure out the task demanded through trial and error and change strategies as needed.

Executive functions are important for successful adaptation and performance in real-life situations. They allow people to initiate and complete tasks and to persevere in the face of challenges. Because the environment can be unpredictable, executive functions are vital to human ability to recognize the significance of unexpected situations and to make alternative plans quickly when unusual events arise and interfere with normal routines. In this way, executive function contributes to success in work and school and allows people to manage the stresses of daily life. Executive functions also enable people to inhibit inappropriate behaviors. People with poor executive functions often have problems interacting with other people since they may say or do things that are bizarre or offensive to others. Most people experience impulses to do or say things that could get them in trouble, such as making a sexually explicit comment to a stranger, commenting negatively on someone's appearance, or insulting an authority figure like a boss or police officer; but most people have no trouble suppressing these urges. When executive functions are impaired, however, these urges may not be suppressed. Executive functions are thus an important component of the ability to fit in socially.

Executive function deficits are associated with a number of psychiatric and developmental disorders, including obsessive-compulsive disorder, Tourette's syndrome, depression, schizophrenia, attention-deficit/hyperactivity disorder, and autism. Executive function deficits also appear to play a role in antisocial behavior. Chronic heavy users of drugs and alcohol show impairments on tests of executive function. Some of these deficits appear to result from heavy substance use, but there is also evidence suggesting that problems with executive functions may contribute to the development of substance use disorders.

Because executive functions govern so many lower-level abilities, there is some controversy about their physiological basis. Nevertheless, most people who study these abilities agree that the frontal lobes of the brain play a major role in executive function. The frontal lobes are the large portions of the brain cortex that lie near the front of the brain. The cortex is the site in the brain where lower level processes like sensation and perception are processed and integrated into thoughts, memories and abilities, and actions are planned and initiated. People with frontal lobe injuries have difficulty with the higher level processing that underlies executive functions. Because of its complexity, the frontal cortex develops more slowly than other parts of the brain, and not surprisingly, many executive functions do not fully develop until adolescence. Some executive functions also appear to decline in old age, and some executive function deficits may be useful in early detection of mild dementia.

Impaired Executive Function Linked to Suicidal Behavior in Elderly. Executive-function impairment is associated with suicide attempts and thoughts in elderly patients with depression and is predictive of behavior disturbance in those with dementia.

More than other dimensions of cognition, executive
function appears to be a key indicator of long-term outcomes in
elderly patients. Impaired executive function has been linked to
greater suicide risk in patients with depression, as well as
worsening behavior disturbance in dementia patients.

In a case-control study conducted by Alexandre Dombrovski,
M.D., and colleagues, 32 people aged 60 or older who had severe
suicidal ideation (with a specific plan, causing them to be
hospitalized) or who had made suicide attempts within the
previous three months, were compared with 32 elderly participants
with matching demographics but who were not suicidal.

Both groups met *DSM-IV* criteria for depression and had similar
scores on the Mini-Mental State Examination. But the suicidal
participants had significantly worse executive function than non-
suicidal ones in the Executive Interview (EXIT25), a 25-item test
that detects left frontal cortical pathology. This difference
in executive function persisted after the authors controlled
for dementia, substance use, medications, or brain injury due to
suicide attempts.

The suicidal participants were also significantly worse in
global cognitive function, measured by the Dementia Rating Scale
and in its attention and memory subscale, but not in
initiation, construction, or the conceptualization subscales. The
study was funded by grants from the National Institutes of
Health, University of Pittsburgh Medical Center, and John A.
Hartford Foundation.

Executive-function impairment in early stages of dementia
was also found to predict more severe behavior disturbance in
patients with dementia, another study reported. Researchers at
Leicester General Hospital in the United Kingdom followed a
group of elderly patients with mild to moderate dementia.

In the 42 dementia patients for whom data were available,
higher scores for executive function on the Cambridge
Examination for Mental Disorders of the Elderly-Revised were

statistically significantly associated with greater behavior disturbance and caregiver distress three to six years later. Global cognitive impairment at baseline, however, was not significantly predictive.

While neither study was randomized or had a large sample size, both add to the growing neuropsychiatry research into the role of prefrontal cortex in certain dimensions and outcomes of mental illness.

"Clearly evident in all of these articles is the substantial importance of cognitive impairments in later life adjustment,...[and] not all cognitive impairments are the same," wrote Philip Harvey, Ph.D., a professor of psychiatry at Emory University School of Medicine, in an accompanying editorial in the journal.

Harvey and both studies' authors acknowledged that medical science still has little knowledge about why and how executive-function impairment is so detrimental to outcomes in not only the elderly, but also in younger patients with mental illness. And even less is known, they said, about whether anything can be done to prevent or mitigate the impairment. They recommended the use of more comprehensive cognitive assessment, especially of executive function, in elderly patients with a variety of conditions.

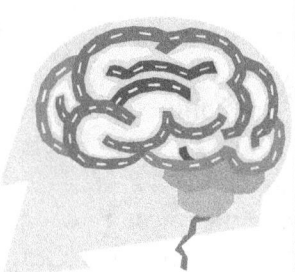

Onset of Dementia

- Early onset: before the age of 60
  - Less than 5% of all cases of AD
  - Strong genetic link
  - Tends to progress more rapidly
- Late onset: after age 60
  - Represents majority of cases

Source: (Mayo Clinic)

What is early onset dementia?

Dementia is the term used to describe the symptoms of a large group of illnesses which cause a progressive decline in a person's mental functioning. It is a broad term which describes a loss of memory, intellect, rationality, social skills, and normal emotional reactions. The term early onset dementia or younger onset dementia is usually used to describe people under the age of sixty five with any form of dementia.

Early onset dementia is a term that covers a range of diseases affecting memory and thinking in people under the age of 65. This group has important medical and social needs that in the past have not always been met. Although most dementias affect people who are elderly, occasionally younger people are diagnosed with dementia. Dementia has been diagnosed in people in their 50's, 40's and even in their 30's. Dementia in younger people is much less common than dementia occurring after the age of 65. For this reason it can be difficult to diagnose and its incidence in the community is still not clear.

The symptoms of early onset dementia are serious. The sense of loss for the person with younger onset dementia and their family can be enormous. Unplanned loss of income, if the main earner was the person with dementia, can be a major problem for the family. The loss of income can be made worse by the loss of the self esteem that usually comes with working, and the loss of a purpose in life. Future plans, perhaps for travel or time with children and grandchildren are no longer viable. Children may react differently to the disease, but are likely to have strong reactions. At a time when they are trying to cope with their own growing up, they find that they also have to cope with a family member who is ill. They may become angry and withdrawn. Some young people may have problems talking with parents because they don't want to worry them or are afraid of making them sad or being an extra burden. They may prefer to talk to people of their own age or to counselors.

Late-onset Alzheimer's disease. This is the most common form of Alzheimer's disease, usually occurring after age 65. Late-onset Alzheimer's disease strikes almost half of all people over the age of 85 and may or may not be hereditary. Late-onset dementia is also called sporadic Alzheimer's disease.

Familial Alzheimer's disease (FAD). This is a form of Alzheimer's disease that is known to be entirely inherited. In affected families, members of at least two generations have had Alzheimer's disease. FAD is extremely rare, accounting for less than 1% of all cases of Alzheimer's disease. It has a much earlier onset (often in the 40s) and can be clearly seen to run in families.

Features Associated with Dementia

- Agitation
- Aggression
- Sleep disturbances
- Apathy (can be misdiagnosed as depression)
- Depression or anxiety
- Personality changes

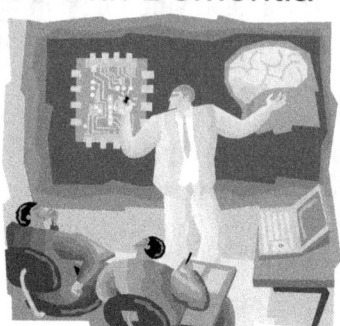

Source: (Health Central)

Definition

Agitation is an unpleasant state of extreme arousal, increased tension, and irritability.

Considerations

Extreme agitation can lead to:

- Confusion.
- Hostility.
- Hyperactivity.

Agitation can come on suddenly or over time. It can last for just a few minutes, or for weeks and even months. Pain, stress, and fever can all increase agitation. Agitation by itself may not be a sign of a health problem. However, if other symptoms occur, it can be a sign of disease.

When agitation lasts for hours and there is changed awareness (altered consciousness), doctors often call this "delirium." Usually this has a medical cause such as alcohol withdrawal or an infection (in elderly adults). Older adults often have delirium while hospitalized.

Causes

Causes of agitation include:

- Alcohol withdrawal.
- Caffeine.
- Cocaine, hallucinogenic drugs, ephedrine.
- Cocaine withdrawal.
- Hyperthyroidism.
- Medical tests that involve injecting a "contrast medium" into the client.
- Nicotine withdrawal.
- Opiate withdrawal.
- Theophylline or other medicines.
- Vitamin B6 deficiency.

Agitation can be associated with:

- Anxiety.
- Bipolar disorder.
- Dementia (such as Alzheimer's disease).
- Depression.
- Schizophrenia.

Home Care

The following can reduce agitation:

- A calm environment.
- Adequate lighting.
- Plenty of sleep.
- Stress-reducing measures.
- Don't restrain an overly-agitated person if possible. This usually worsens the problem.
- Communicating your feelings is important.

When to Contact a Medical Professional

Contact a health care provider if the client experience prolonged or severe agitation, especially if there are other unexplained symptoms.

What to Expect at an Office Visit

A health care provider will take a medical history and do a physical examination.

To help better understand the agitation, s/he may ask the client the following questions:

- Are you more talkative than usual or do you feel pressure to keep talking?
- Do you find yourself doing purposeless activities (e.g., pacing, hand wringing)?
- Are you extremely restless?
- Are you trembling or twitching?
- Time pattern.
- Was the agitation a short episode?
- Is the agitation persistent?
- How long did it last -- for how many day(s)?
- Aggravating factors.
- Does the agitation seem to be triggered by reminders of a traumatic event?
- Did you notice anything else that may have triggered agitation?
- Do you take any medications, especially steroids or thyroid medicine?
- How much alcohol do you drink?
- How much caffeine do you drink?
- Do you use any drugs, such as cocaine, narcotics, or "speed" (amphetamines)?
- What other symptoms do you have?
- Is there confusion, memory loss, hyperactivity, or hostility (these symptoms can play an important role in diagnosis).

Aggression

Most patients with mental disorders are not aggressive. Nonetheless, epidemiological evidence points to an increased risk for violence among individuals with a mental disorder compared with the general population. This article reviews this evidence and provides a framework for the assessment and treatment of these individuals.

Aggressive behavior in patients with psychiatric disorders has many possible causes. Probably the most important causes are the presence of comorbid substance abuse, dependence, and intoxication. In addition, the disease process itself may produce hallucinations and delusions, which may provoke violence. Often, poor impulse control related to neuropsychiatric deficits may facilitate the discharge of aggressive tendencies. Finally, underlying personality characteristics, such as antisocial personality traits, also may influence the use of violent acts as a means to achieve certain goals. Environmental factors that are associated with aggressive behavior include a chaotic or unstable home or hospital situation, which may encourage maladaptive aggressive behaviors.

Terms such as aggression, violence, crime, and hostility are observed in medical literature. Aggression is used for both humans and animals. In humans, aggression can denote verbal aggression, physical aggression against objects, or physical aggression against people. At times, aggression towards oneself (self-mutilation, suicidal gestures or acts) is included in the definition. Violence is used only when describing human behavior and denotes physical aggression by one person against another. Crime is defined as the intentional violation of criminal law. Hostility is a loosely defined term and can refer to aggression, irritability, suspicion, uncooperativeness, or jealousy.

Assessment

Client assessment involves:

1. The gathering of information about past and current behavior from the client, health care providers, family, and friends.
2. A review of past treatment (successful and unsuccessful).
3. A clinical examination of the client over time.

In the assessment of a client who is acutely agitated and whose history is unknown, attempts are made to rule out somatic conditions that require emergency treatment. Delirium is a medical emergency. Once the client is under behavioral control, further medical and psychiatric workups can be accomplished.

Mechanical restraints may be necessary to prevent agitated patients from injuring themselves or others while the medical workup is being conducted. For patients who are acutely agitated and for whom the episode is one of many, the acute episode is managed, and, subsequently, time is devoted to strategies designed to reduce the intensity and frequency of episodes.

Included in a physical examination should be a thorough mental status examination. Key elements include an assessment of affect and thought content, especially hallucinations, delusions, suicidal ideation, and homicidal ideation. An assessment of orientation and memory is also crucial for establishing a differential diagnosis. Disorientation may be the first clue that an underlying somatic condition is altering the client's mental status.

Care must be taken to not miss comorbid conditions that may manifest as acute intoxication or withdrawal, such as alcohol or sedative abuse or dependence. A concomitant seizure disorder may complicate the clinical picture, especially if neuroleptic therapy appears to worsen the condition. Adverse drug effects, such as akathisia, may serve as stimuli for striking out. Antisocial personality traits may be the most important factor in some instances of client violence in which goal-directed behavior, such as extortion of money or cigarettes, is evident.

The principal elements of the non-pharmacological management of aggressive behavior include the following:
- Assess the environment for potential dangers (e.g., objects that can be thrown or used as a weapon).
- Assess the physical demeanor of the client (e.g., many patients make a fist before punching or kicking).
- Know where the client is at all times (e.g., do not turn your back to the client; do not leave the client alone and therefore unobserved).
- Take verbal threats seriously.
- Remain several feet away to avoid crowding the client.
- Clear the area of other patients.

- Summon additional help (a "show of force" or a "show of concern"); this is not a time for heroics.
- Remain calm, maintain a confident and competent demeanor, and attempt to deescalate by engaging the client in conversation.
- Avoid arguments between staff members in front of the client.
- If restraints are necessary, have at least 4 people available.

Medications are often used to manage agitated behavior. These include benzodiazepines (e.g., lorazepam) and antipsychotics (e.g., haloperidol). The US Food and Drug Administration (FDA) has approved new intramuscular formulations of second-generation antipsychotics that can be used to calm agitated patients. Ziprasidone intramuscular is approved for use in agitation associated with schizophrenia, and olanzapine intramuscular and aripiprazole intramuscular are approved for use in agitation associated with either schizophrenia or bipolar mania. In general, intramuscular injection has a faster onset of action than oral administration; however, a client may calm down readily after an oral dose because he or she realizes that action has been taken and help is being provided. Sublingual administration may have a faster onset of action than oral ingestion and has the added advantage of distracting the agitated client while the pill is dissolving.

Sleep Disturbances
The most common sleep disorders include:
- Insomnia: Continuously having difficulty in falling asleep and sleep maintenance.
- Bruxism: Involuntarily grinding or clenching of the teeth while sleeping.
- Delayed sleep phase syndrome (DSPS): inability to awaken and fall asleep at socially acceptable times but no problem with sleep maintenance, a disorder of circadian rhythms. Other such disorders are advanced sleep phase syndrome (ASPS) and Non-24-hour sleep-wake syndrome (Non-24), both much less common than DSPS.

- Hypopnea syndrome: Abnormally shallow breathing or slow respiratory rate while sleeping.
- Narcolepsy: Excessive daytime sleepiness, often culminating in falling asleep spontaneously and unwillingly at inappropriate times. Cataplexy, a sudden weakness in the motor muscles that could result in collapse to the floor is also common.
- Night terror, *Pavor nocturnus*, sleep terror disorder: abrupt awakening from sleep with behavior consistent with terror.
- Parasomnias: Disruptive sleep-related events involving inappropriate actions during sleep stages - sleep walking and night-terrors are examples.
- Periodic limb movement disorder (PLMD): Sudden involuntary movement of arms and/or legs during sleep, for example kicking the legs. Also known as nocturnal myoclonus. See also Hypnic jerk, which is not a disorder.
- Rapid eye movement behavior disorder (RBD): Acting out violent or dramatic dreams while in REM sleep.
- Restless legs syndrome (RLS): An irresistible urge to move legs. RLS sufferers often also have PLMD.
- Situational circadian rhythm sleep disorders: shift work sleep disorder (SWSD) and jet lag.
- Obstructive sleep apnea: Obstruction of the airway during sleep, causing lack of sufficient deep sleep; often accompanied by snoring. Central sleep apnea is less common.
- Sleep paralysis is characterized by temporary paralysis of the body shortly before or after sleep. Sleep paralysis may be accompanied
  by visual, auditory, or tactile hallucinations. Not a disorder unless severe. Often seen as part of narcolepsy.
- Sleepwalking or *somnambulism*: Engaging in activities that are normally associated with wakefulness (such as eating or dressing), which may include walking, without the conscious knowledge of the subject.

Treatments for sleep disorders generally can be grouped into four categories:

- Behavioral/ psychotherapeutic treatments.
- Rehabilitation/management.
- Medications.
- Other somatic treatments.

None of these general approaches is sufficient for all patients with sleep disorders. Rather, the choice of a specific treatment depends on the client's diagnosis, medical and psychiatric history, and preferences, as well as the expertise of the treating clinician. Often, behavioral/psychotherapeutic and pharmacological approaches are not incompatible and can effectively be combined to maximize therapeutic benefits. Management of sleep disturbances that are secondary to mental, medical, or substance abuse disorders should focus on the underlying conditions.

Medications and somatic treatments may provide the most rapid symptomatic relief from some sleep disturbances. Some disorders, such as narcolepsy, are best treated pharmacologically. Others, such as chronic and primary insomnia, may be more amenable to behavioral interventions, with more durable results.

Special equipment may be required for treatment of several disorders such as obstructive apnea, the circadian rhythm disorders, and bruxism. In these cases, when severe, an acceptance of living with the disorder, however well managed, is often necessary.

Apathy
The absence or suppression of passion, emotion, or excitement. A lack of interest in or concern for things that others find moving or exciting. Treatment similar to those for depression.

Source: (eMedicine Health)
Depression
Overview
Throughout the course of our lives, we all experience episodes of unhappiness, sadness, or grief. Often, when a loved one dies or we suffer a personal tragedy or difficulty such as divorce or loss of a

job, we may feel depressed (some people call this "the blues").
Most of us are able to cope with these and other types of stressful
events.

Over a period of days or weeks, the majority of us are able to
return to our normal activities. But when these feelings of sadness
and other symptoms make it hard for us to get through the day, and
when the symptoms last for more than a couple of weeks, we may
have what is called clinical depression. The term "clinical
depression" is usually used to distinguish "true" depression from
the blues.

Clinical depression is not just grief or sadness. It is an illness that
can challenge your ability to perform even routine daily activities.
At its worst, depression may lead to contemplate or commit
suicide. Depression represents a burden for the whole family.
Sometimes that burden can seem overwhelming.

There are several different types of depression (mood disorders
that include depressive symptoms):
- **Major depression** is a change in mood that lasts for weeks
  or months. It is one of the most severe types of depression.
  It usually involves a low or irritable mood and/or a loss of
  interest or pleasure in usual activities. It interferes with
  one's normal functioning and often includes physical
  symptoms. A person may experience only one episode, but
  often there are repeated episodes over an individual's
  lifetime.

- **Dysthymia** is less severe than major depression but usually
  goes on for a longer period, often several years. There are
  usually periods of feeling fairly normal between episodes
  of low mood. The symptoms usually do not completely
  disrupt one's normal activities.

- **Seasonal depression**, which medical professionals
  call seasonal affective disorder, or SAD, is depression that
  occurs only at a certain time of the year, usually winter. It

is sometimes called "winter blues." Although it is predictable, it can be very severe.

- **Adjustment disorder** is distress that occurs in relation to a stressful life event. It is usually an isolated reaction that resolves when the <u>stress</u> passes. Although it may be accompanied by a depressed mood, it is not considered a depressive disorder.

Some people believe that depression is "normal" in people who are elderly, have other health problems, have setbacks or other tragedies, or have bad life situations. On the contrary, clinical depression is always abnormal and always requires attention from a medical or mental-health professional. The good news is that depression can be diagnosed and treated effectively in most people. The biggest barrier to overcoming depression is recognizing that someone is depressed and seeking appropriate treatment.

Source: (Help Guide.org)
Treatment of Depression
Self-Care at Home
Make lifestyle changes and choices that will help the client through the rough times and may prevent depression from returning:

- Try to identify and focus on activities which make the client feel better. It is important the s/he does things for themselves. Don't isolate or allow the client to isolate themselves. Encourage the client to take part in activities even when they may not want to. Such activity may actually make them feel better.
- Encourage them to talk with friends and family and consider joining a support group. Communicating and discussing feelings is an integral part of treatment and will help with recovery.
- Try to maintain a positive outlook. Having a good attitude can be beneficial.

- Regular exercise and proper diet are essential to good health. Exercise has been found to increase the levels of the body's own natural antidepressants called endorphins.
- Ensure the client gets enough rest and maintain a regular sleeping pattern.
- Avoid drinking alcohol or using any illicit substances.

Personality Changes

These are numerous and can be significant. All of the above and others will lead to some form of personality change. Knowing the client; observing their daily routine; and regular interaction with them will alert an observant caregiver to abnormal, sudden, or significant changes in personality.

Features Associated with Dementia

- Behavioral disinhibition
- Impaired insight
- Hallucinations (visual more common than auditory)
- Delusions (often paranoid or persecutory)

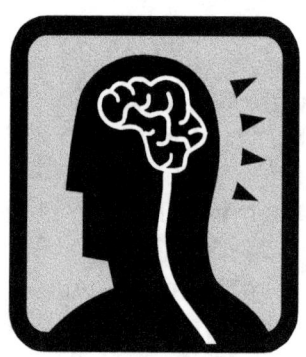

Source: (Wikipedia)

Behavioral Disinhibition

Individuals who show disinhibited behavior tend to have this as part of a cluster of challenging behaviors including verbal aggression, physical aggression, socially inappropriate behavior, sexual disinhibition, wandering, and repetitive behavior.

Disinhibited behavior occurs when people do not follow the social rules about what or where to say or do something. People who are disinhibited may come across as rude, tactless, or even offensive. For example, a person with a brain injury may make a comment about how ugly another person is, or a person with dementia may have lost their social manners and look as though they are deliberately harassing another person.

Sexually disinhibited persons may inappropriately flirt with someone, make sexual comments for example, and say things like 'you look hot', or 'I want to touch your breasts', or 'I want to feel your cock'. A person might expose themselves such as taking off part or all their clothes in public. They may unexpectedly fondle themselves or masturbate in public. They may touch other people on their face, arms, legs, buttocks, or genitals.

Source: (Medline Plus)
Hallucinations
Definition
Hallucinations involve sensing things that aren't there while a person is awake and conscious.

Considerations
Common hallucinations include:
- Feeling a crawling sensation on the skin.
- Hearing voices when no one has spoken.
- Seeing patterns, lights, beings, or objects that aren't there.
- Hallucinations related to smell or taste are rare.

Many recreational drugs, including drugs such as LSD and certain strong types of marijuana, may cause hallucinations. Hallucinations related to these drugs tend to involve seeing things, and may include patterns or haloes around lights. People who have such visual hallucinations after taking drugs usually know that their perception is distorted.

Hearing things (auditory hallucinations) is more common in psychotic conditions such as schizophrenia, although it may sometimes occur with high doses of cocaine, amphetamines, or other stimulants. High doses of stimulant drugs can make one feel as though there are bugs crawling on or just under the skin.

In some cases, hallucinations may be normal. For example, hearing the voice of, or briefly seeing, a loved one who has recently died can be a part of the grieving process.

When to Contact a Medical Professional
A person who begins to hallucinate and is detached from reality should get checked by a health care professional right away, because many medical conditions that can cause hallucinations may quickly become emergencies. A person who is hallucinating may become nervous, paranoid, and frightened, and should not be left alone.

Call your health care provider, go to the emergency room, or call the local emergency number (such as 911) if someone appears to be hallucinating and is unable to tell hallucinations from reality.

What to Expect at Your Office Visit
The health care provider will do a physical examination and take a medical history. Blood may be drawn for testing.

Medical history questions may include the following:
- Do you hear a voice?
- Do you see something?
- Are there sensations of feeling something or being touched?
- How long have there been hallucinations?
- When did the hallucinations first appear?
- Do the hallucinations occur just before or after sleep?
- Has there been a recent death or other emotional event?
- What medications are being taken?
- Use of alcohol?
- Use of illegal drugs?
- Are the hallucinations related to a traumatic event?
- Is there agitation?
- Is there confusion?

- Is there a fever?
- Is there a headache?
- Is there vomiting?

Source: (Encyclopedia of Mental Disorder)
Delusions
A delusion is a belief that is clearly false and that indicates an abnormality in the affected person's content of thought. The false belief is not accounted for by the person's cultural or religious background or his or her level of intelligence. The key feature of a delusion is the degree to which the person is convinced that the belief is true. A person with a delusion will hold firmly to the belief regardless of evidence to the contrary. Delusions can be difficult to distinguish from overvalued ideas, which are unreasonable ideas that a person holds, but the affected person has at least some level of doubt as to its truthfulness. A person with a delusion is absolutely convinced that the delusion is real.

Depression

- **Onset**: rapid
- **Precipitants**: psycho-social (not organic)
- **Duration**: less than 3 months to presentation
- **Mood**: depressed, anxious
- **Behavior**: decreased activity or agitation
- **Cognition**: unimpaired or poor responses
- **Somatic symptoms**: fatigue, lethargy, sleep, appetite disruption
- **Course**: rapid resolution with treatment, may precede Alzheimer's disease

---

Source: (Depression guide)
Some people say that depression feels like a black curtain of despair coming down over their lives. Many people feel like they have no energy and can't concentrate. Others feel irritable all the

time for no apparent reason. The symptoms vary from person to person, but when a client feels "down" for more than two weeks, and these feelings are interfering with his/her daily life, they may be clinically depressed.

Most people who have gone through one episode of depression will, sooner or later, have another one. They may begin to feel some of the symptoms of depression several weeks before they develop a full-blown episode of depression. Learning to recognize these early triggers or symptoms and working with their doctor will help to keep the depression from worsening.

Most people with depression never seek help, even though the majority will respond to treatment. Treating depression is especially important because it affects the whole family. Some people with depression may try to harm themselves in the mistaken belief that the feelings will never change. Depression is a treatable illness.

Life with Depression

Working with a doctor, one can learn to manage depression. It may be necessary to try a few different medications to find the one that works. A doctor may also recommend seeing a therapist and/or make certain lifestyle changes. Change will not come overnight—but with the right treatment, depression can be prevented from overshadowing life.

Treatment Tips

Antidepressant medications work for many people—they can make some feel better, and can improve or completely relieve symptoms. But sometimes people have unrealistic fears or expectations about them. Some hope to feel better overnight; others worry that medications will change their personalities in ways they won't like. Both extremes are unlikely. The first step towards getting better and staying better is to take medication exactly as prescribed by a doctor.

Here are some treatment tips:
- It takes time for antidepressants to work. Although one may start to feel better within a couple of weeks, the full antidepressant effect may not be seen for several weeks. It is important to be patient and give the medicine a chance to work.
- Once you feel better, it is important to keep taking your antidepressant for as long as your doctor tells you to. Continued use, if recommended by your doctor, can help lower your chances of becoming depressed again in the future.
- Although some people only become depressed once, others—especially those who have been depressed before or have several risk factors—may need longer term treatment with medication.
- If a client or the family wants to stop, do so after discussing this with their doctor.

Like many drugs, depression medications can cause side effects and interact with foods or other medications. Inform the doctor about any medical conditions and other medicines being used. If the client experiences drug side effects, contact the doctor right away.

Diet for Depression
Trying to find a diet to ease depression? Unfortunately, there's no specific diet that works for depression. No studies have been done that indicate a particular eating plan can ease symptoms of clinical depression.

Still, while certain diets or foods may not ease depression (or put you instantly in a better mood), they may help as part of an overall treatment for depression. There's more and more research indicating that, in some ways, food and mood are connected.

Source: (WebMD)
How can my diet affect my depression?
Dietary changes can bring about changes in your brain structure, both chemically and physiologically. Those changes can improve mood and mental outlook. Here are 10 tips for eating if you or a loved one is recovering from clinical depression.

1. Eat a diet high in nutrients
Nutrients in foods support the body's repair, growth, and wellness. Nutrients we all need include vitamins, minerals, carbohydrates, protein, and even a small amount of fat. A deficiency in any of these nutrients leads to our bodies not working at full capacity – and can even cause illness.

2. Fill the plate with essential antioxidants
Damaging molecules called free radicals are produced in our bodies during normal body functions – and these free radicals contribute to aging and dysfunction. Antioxidants such as beta-carotene and vitamins C and E combat the effects of free radicals. Antioxidants have been shown to tie up these free radicals and take away their destructive power.
Studies show that the brain is particularly at risk for free radical damage. Although there's no way to stop free radicals completely, we can reduce their destructive effect on the body by eating foods high in powerful antioxidants, including:
- **Sources of beta-carotene:** apricots, broccoli, cantaloupe, carrots, collards, peaches, pumpkin, spinach, sweet potato.
- **Sources of vitamin C:** blueberries, broccoli, grapefruit, kiwi, oranges, peppers, potatoes, strawberries, tomato.
- **Sources of vitamin E:** margarine, nuts and seeds, vegetable oils, wheat germ.

3. Eat "smart" carbohydrates for a calming effect
The connection between carbohydrates and mood is linked to the mood-boosting brain chemical, serotonin. We know that eating foods high in carbohydrates (breads, cereal, and pasta) raises the level of serotonin in the brain. When serotonin levels rise, we feel a calming effect with less anxiety.

So don't shun carbs – just make smart choices. Limit sugary foods and opt for smart carbohydrates, such as whole grains, fruits, vegetables, and legumes, which all contribute healthy carbs as well as fiber.

4. Eat protein-rich foods to boost alertness

Foods rich in protein, like turkey, tuna, or chicken, are rich in an amino acid called tyrosine. Tyrosine boosts levels of the brain chemicals dopamine and norepinephrine. This boost helps one feel alert and makes it easier to concentrate. Try to include a protein source in your diet several times a day, especially when a clear mind and energy boost is needed.

Good sources of protein foods that boost alertness: beans and peas, lean beef, low-fat cheese, fish, milk, poultry, soy products, yogurt.

5. Eat a Mediterranean diet

The Mediterranean diet is a balanced, healthy eating pattern that includes plenty of fruits, nuts, vegetables, cereals, legumes, and fish. All of these are important sources of nutrients linked to preventing depression.

A recent Spanish study, using data from 4,211 men and 5,459 women, found that rates of depression tended to increase in men -- especially smokers -- as folate intake decreased. The same increase occurred for women -- especially those who smoked or were physically active -- but with a decreased intake of another B-vitamin: B12. This wasn't the first study to discover an association between these two vitamins and depression. Researchers wonder whether poor nutrient intake leads to depression or whether depression leads people to eat a poor diet.

Folate is found in Mediterranean diet staples like legumes, nuts, many fruits, and particularly dark green vegetables. B12 can be found in all lean and low-fat animal products, such as fish and low-fat dairy products.

6. Get plenty of vitamin D

Vitamin D increases levels of serotonin in the brain. Researchers, though, are unsure how much vitamin D is ideal. There are individual differences based on where one lives, the time of year, skin type, and level of sun exposure. Researchers from the University of Toronto noticed that people who were suffering from depression, particularly those with seasonal affective disorder, tended to improve as their levels of vitamin D in the body increased over the normal course of a year. The recommendation is to try to get about 600 international units (IU) of vitamin D a day from food if possible.

7. Select selenium-rich foods

Selenium is a mineral that is essential to good health. In a small study from Texas Tech University, supplementation of 200 micrograms a day for seven weeks improved mild and moderate depression in 16 elderly participants. Other studies have also reported an association between low selenium intakes and poorer moods.

It is possible to take in too much selenium so that it becomes toxic. But this is unlikely if it is gotten from foods rather than supplements, and it can't hurt to make sure the client eats foods that help them meet the recommended intake for selenium, which is 55 micrograms a day. The good news is that foods rich in selenium are foods oen should be eating anyway. They include:

- Beans and legumes.
- Lean meat (lean pork and beef, skinless chicken and turkey).
- Low-fat dairy products.
- Nuts and seeds (particularly Brazil nuts).
- Seafood (oysters, clams, sardines, crab, saltwater fish, and freshwater fish).
- Whole grains (whole-grain pasta, brown rice, oatmeal, etc.).

8. Include omega-3 fatty acids in the diet

We know that omega-3 fatty acids have innumerable health benefits. Recently, scientists have revealed that a deficit of omega-3 fatty acids is associated with depression. In one study, researchers determined that societies that eat a small amount of omega-3 fatty acids have a higher prevalence of major depressive disorder than societies that get ample omega-3 fatty acids. Other epidemiological studies show that people who infrequently eat fish, which is a rich source of omega-3 fatty acids, are more likely to suffer from depression.

- **Sources of omega-3 fatty acids:** fatty fish (anchovy, mackerel, salmon, sardines, shad, and tuna), flaxseed, and nuts.
- **Sources alpha-linolenic acid (another type of omega-3 fatty acid):** flaxseed, canola oil, soybean oil, walnuts, and dark green leafy vegetables.

9. Watch lifestyle habits

Many people who are depressed also have problems with alcohol and/or drugs. Not only can alcohol and drugs interfere with mood, sleep, and motivation, they can also affect the effectiveness of your depression medications. In addition, drinks and foods containing caffeine can trigger anxiety and make it difficult to sleep at night. Cutting out caffeine or stopping caffeine after noon each day can also help one get a better night's sleep.

10. Stay at a healthy weight

Findings published in the journal of *Clinical Psychology: Science and Practice*, show a link between obesity and depression, indicating that people who are obese may be more likely to become depressed. In addition, according to this study, people who are depressed are more likely to become obese. Researchers believe the link between obesity and depression may result from physiological changes that occur in the immune system and hormones with depression. Consult a doctor about healthy ways to manage it with diet and exercise.

Exercise and Depression
Want to learn more about exercise and depression? Many studies indicate that people who exercise regularly benefit with a positive boost in mood and lower rates of depression.

What are the psychological benefits of exercise with depression?
Improved self-esteem is a key psychological benefit of regular physical activity. When exercising, the body releases chemicals called endorphins. These endorphins interact with the receptors in the brain that reduce the perception of pain.

Endorphins also trigger a positive feeling in the body, similar to that of morphine. For example, the feeling that follows a run or workout is often described as "euphoric." That feeling, known as a "runner's high," can be accompanied by a positive and energizing outlook on life.

Endorphins act as analgesics, which mean they diminish the perception of pain. They also act as sedatives. They are manufactured in your brain, spinal cord, and many other parts of your body and are released in response to brain chemicals called neurotransmitters. The neuron receptors endorphins bind to are the same ones that bind some pain medicines. However, unlike with morphine, the activation of these receptors by the body's endorphins does not lead to addiction or dependence.
Regular exercise has been proven to help:
- Reduce stress.
- Ward off anxiety and feelings of depression.
- Boost self-esteem.
- Improve sleep.

Exercise also has these added health benefits:
- It strengthens the heart.
- It increases energy levels.
- It lowers blood pressure.
- It improves muscle tone and strength.
- It strengthens and builds bones.

- It helps reduce body fat.
- It makes one look fit and healthy.

Is exercise a treatment for clinical depression?
Research has shown that exercise is an effective but often underused treatment for mild to moderate depression.

Source: (The Clements Clinic)
Do particular types of exercise help depression?
It appears that any form of exercise can help depression. Some examples of moderate exercise include:
- Biking.
- Dancing.
- Gardening.
- Golf (walking instead of using the cart).
- Housework, especially sweeping, mopping, or vacuuming.
- Jogging at a moderate pace.
- Low-impact aerobics.
- Playing tennis.
- Swimming.
- Walking.
- Yard work, especially mowing or raking.
- Yoga.

Because strong social support is important for those with depression, joining a group exercise class may be beneficial. Or exercise with a close friend or partner. One will benefit from the physical activity and emotional comfort, knowing that others are supportive.

Do I need to check with my doctor before starting an exercise program?
For most people, it is okay to start an exercise program without checking with a health care provider. However, if the client has not exercised in a while, or has a medical condition such as diabetes or heart disease, contact their health care provider before starting an exercise program.

Delirium Definition

- Disturbance of consciousness
  - i.e., reduced clarity of awareness of environment with reduced ability to focus, sustain, or shift attention
- Change in cognition (memory, orientation, language, perception)
- Development over short period (hours to days), tends to fluctuate

Source: (Algiakrishnan)

Delirium or acute confusion state is a transient global disorder of cognition. The condition is a medical emergency associated with increased morbidity and mortality rates. Early diagnosis and resolution of symptoms are correlated with the most favorable outcomes. Therefore, it must be treated as a medical emergency.

Delirium is not a disease but a syndrome with multiple causes that result in a similar constellation of symptoms. Delirium is defined as a transient, usually reversible, cause of cerebral dysfunction and manifests clinically with a wide range of neuropsychiatric abnormalities. The clinical hallmarks are decreased attention span and a waxing and waning type of confusion.

Delirium often is unrecognized or misdiagnosed and commonly is mistaken for dementia, depression, mania, an acute schizophrenic reaction, or part of old age (patients who are elderly are expected to become confused in the hospital).

The word delirium is derived from the Latin term meaning "off the track." This syndrome was reported during Hippocrates' time, and, in 1813, Sutton described delirium tremens. Later, Wernicke described the encephalopathy that bears his name.

Pathophysiology
Based on the state of arousal, 3 types of delirium are described. Hyperactive delirium is observed in patients in a state of alcohol withdrawal or intoxication with to phencyclidine (PCP), amphetamine, and lysergic acid diethylamide (LSD). Hypoactive delirium is observed in patients in states of hepatic encephalopathy and hypercapnia. In mixed delirium, individuals display daytime sedation with nocturnal agitation and behavioral problems.

The mechanism of delirium still is not fully understood. Delirium results from a wide variety of structural or physiological insults. The neuropathogenesis of delirium has been studied in patients with hepatic encephalopathy and alcohol withdrawal. Research in these areas still is limited. The main hypothesis is reversible impairment of cerebral oxidative metabolism and multiple neurotransmitter abnormalities. The following observations support the hypothesis of multiple neurotransmitter abnormalities. The diagnosis of delirium is clinical. No single test is successful. Obtaining a thorough history is essential.

Because delirious patients often are confused and unable to provide accurate information, getting a detailed history from family, caregivers, and nursing staff is particularly important. Nursing notes can be very helpful for documentation of episodes of disorientation, abnormal behavior, and hallucinations. Learning to record accurate and specific findings in mental status as well as the particular time the finding was observed is imperative for the staff. Staff should not just report "he was confused."

Delirium always should be suspected when an acute or subacute deterioration in behavior, cognition, or function occurs, especially in patients who are elderly, demented, or depressed. Patients may have visual hallucinations or persecutory delusions as well as grandiose delusions. Some patients with delirium also may become suicidal or homicidal. Therefore, they should not be left unattended or alone.

Delirium is mistaken for dementia or depression, especially when patients are quiet or withdrawn. However, by *Diagnostic and Statistical Manual of Mental Disorders, Fourth Edition, Text Revision (DSM-IV-TR)* criteria, dementia cannot be diagnosed with certainty when delirium is present. Health professionals can do Mini-Mental Status Exam (MMSE), depression assessment screening using *DSM-IV-TR* criteria, or the Geriatric Depression Scale (GDS). They can also assess for suicidal and homicidal risk if necessary. Health professionals can directly ask patients about suicidal or homicidal ideation (thoughts), intent, and plan.

Depression symptoms are commonly seen with delirium. In a recent study, patients having symptoms of dysphoric mood and hopelessness are at risk for incident delirium while in the hospital. On the other hand, hypoactive delirium may be mistaken for depression. Up to 42% of patients referred to psychiatry services for suspected depressive illness in the hospital may have delirium. Screening for depression in the presence of delirium is quite challenging.

Delirium is a common cause for psychotic symptoms, bizarre delusions, abnormal behavior, and thought disorders. Agitated patients are at risk for violent and abnormal behavior and in rare circumstances, agitation can lead to attempts of homicide.

The mental status is a bedside or interview assessment that dramatically fluctuates. It includes the client's appearance, affect (mood), thoughts (especially the presence of hallucinations and delusions), inquiry into self-destructive behavior, homicidal behavior, judgment and, in this diagnosis, orientation, immediate, recent, and long-term memory.

Main Symptoms
- Clouding of consciousness.
- Difficulty maintaining or shifting attention.
- Disorientation.
- Illusions.
- Hallucinations.
- Fluctuating levels of consciousness.

Symptoms tend to fluctuate over the course of the day, with some improvement in the daytime and maximum disturbance at night. Reversal of the sleep-wake cycle is common.

- Neurological symptoms.
- Dysphasia.
- Dysarthria.
- Tremor.
- Asterixis in hepatic encephalopathy and uremia.
- Motor abnormalities.
- Patients with delirium who are hyperactive have an increased state of arousal, psychomotor abnormalities, and hyper-vigilance. In contrast, patients with delirium who are hypoactive are withdrawn, less active, and sleepy.
- Hypoactive delirium sometimes is misdiagnosed as dementia or depression. Mixed states also occur.
- In patients who are elderly, delirium often is the presenting symptom of an underlying illness.

Physical
A careful and complete physical examination including a mental status examination is necessary. Testing vital signs such as temperature, pulse, blood pressure, and respiration is mandatory.

Patients have difficulty sustaining attention, problems in orientation and short-term memory, poor insight, and impaired judgment. Key elements here are fluctuating levels of consciousness.

Impaired attention can be assessed with bedside tests that require sustained attention to a task that has not been memorized, such as reciting the days of the week or months of the year backwards, counting backwards from 20, or doing serial subtraction.

DSM-IV-TR **diagnostic criteria for delirium**:
Disturbance of consciousness (i.e., reduced clarity of awareness of the environment) occurs, with reduced ability to focus, sustain, or shift attention. Change in cognition (e.g., memory deficit,

disorientation, language disturbance, perceptual disturbance) occurs that is not better accounted for by a preexisting, established, or evolving dementia.

The disturbance develops over a short period (usually hours to days) and tends to fluctuate during the course of the day. Evidence from the history, physical examination, or laboratory findings is present that indicates the disturbance is caused by a direct physiologic consequence of a general medical condition, an intoxicating substance, medication use, or more than one cause.

Other diagnostic instruments are the Delirium Symptom Interview (DSI) and the Confusion Assessment Method (CAM). Delirium symptom severity can be assessed by the Delirium Rating Scale (DRS) and the Memorial Delirium Assessment Scale (MDAS).

Delirium

- Susceptibility may be symptom of early dementia, or delirium may predispose to later dementia

- Predisposing factors - age, infections, dementia

Features	Delirium	Dementia
Onset	Acute	Insidious
Course	Fluctuating	Progressive
Duration	Days to weeks	Months to years
Consciousness	Altered	Clear
Attention	Impaired	Normal, except for severe dementia
Psychomotor changes	Increased or decreased	Often normal
Reversibility	Usually	Rarely

Source: (Algiakrishnan)

Causes

Almost any medical illness, intoxication, or medication can cause delirium. Often, delirium is multifactorial in etiology, and the physician treating the delirium should investigate each cause contributing to it. Medications are the most common reversible cause of delirium.

DSM-IV-TR classification of delirium :
- Delirium due to general medical condition.
- Substance intoxication delirium.
- Substance withdrawal delirium.
- Delirium due to multiple etiologies.
- Delirium not otherwise specified.

Some of the other common reversible causes include the following:
- Hypoxia.
- Hypoglycemia.
- Hyperthermia.
- Anticholinergic delirium.
- Alcohol or sedative withdrawal.

Other causes of delirium include the following:
- Infections.
- Metabolic abnormalities.
- Structural lesions of the brain.
- Postoperative states.

Miscellaneous causes, such as sensory deprivation, sleep deprivation, fecal impaction, urinary retention, and change of environment. In the elderly, medications at therapeutic doses and levels can cause delirium.

Although numerous risk factors have been described, a recent study identified 5 important independent risk factors:
- Use of physical restraints.
- Malnutrition.
- Use of a bladder catheter.
- Any iatrogenic event.
- Use of 3 or more medications.

Dementia is one of the strongest most consistent risk factors. Underlying dementia is observed in 25-50% of patients. The presence of dementia increases the risk of delirium 2-3 times. Low educational level, which may be an indicator of low cognitive reserve, is associated with increased vulnerability to delirium.

Dysphoric mood and hopelessness are also risk factors for incident delirium:

- Structural changes.
- Closed head injury or cerebral hemorrhage.
- Cerebrovascular accidents, such as cerebral infarction, subarachnoid hemorrhage, and hypertensive encephalopathy.
- Primary or metastatic brain tumors.
- Brain abscess.

Metabolic causes:

- Fluid and electrolyte abnormalities, acid-base disturbances, and hypoxia.
- Hypoglycemia.
- Hepatic or renal failure.
- Vitamin deficiency states (especially thiamine and cyanocobalamin).
- Endocrinopathies associated with the thyroid and parathyroid.

Hypoperfusion states:

- Shock.
- Congestive heart failure.
- Cardiac arrhythmias.
- Anemias.

Infectious causes:

- CNS infections such as meningitis.
- Encephalitis.
- HIV-related brain infections.
- Septicemia.

- Pneumonia.
- Urinary tract infections.

Toxic causes:
- Substance intoxication - Alcohol, heroin, cannabis, PCP, and LSD.
- Medication-induced delirium.
- Anticholinergics (Benadryl, tricyclic antidepressants).
- Narcotics (meperidine).
- Sedative hypnotics (benzodiazepines).
- Histamine-2 (H2) blockers (cimetidine).
- Corticosteroids.
- Centrally acting antihypertensives (methyldopa, reserpine).
- Anti-Parkinson drugs (levodopa).
- Substance withdrawal from alcohol, opioids, and benzodiazepines.

Other causes:
- Postictal state.
- Unfamiliar environment.

Eyes, Ears, Environment

- Sensory deficits may contribute to appearance of patient being demented
- Central Auditory Processing Deficits (CAPD)
- Hearing problems are socially isolating
- Visual problems are difficult to accommodate by a demented patient, e.g. to do cataract operation
- Nutritional deficiencies (e.g. tea & toast syndrome)

Source: (Schminky, 1999)

Central Auditory Processing Disorders - Overview of Assessment & Management Practices

Hearing is a complex process that is often taken for granted. As sounds strike the eardrum, the sounds (acoustic signals) begin to undergo a series of transformations through which the acoustic signals are changed into neural signals. These neural signals are then passed from the ear through complicated neural networks to various parts of the brain for additional analysis, and ultimately, recognition or comprehension. For most of us, when someone talks about hearing abilities, we think primarily of the processing that occurs in the ear; that is, the ability to detect the presence of sound. Likewise, when someone is described as having a hearing loss, we assume that this individual has lost all or part of the ability to detect the presence of sound. However, the ability to detect the presence of sounds is only one part of the processing that occurs within the auditory system.

There are many individuals who have no trouble detecting the presence of sound, but who have other types of auditory difficulties (e.g., difficulties understanding conversations in noisy environments, problems following complex directions, difficulty learning new vocabulary words or foreign languages) that can affect their ability to develop normal language skills, succeed academically, or communicate effectively. Often these individuals are not recognized as having hearing difficulties because they do not have trouble detecting the presence of sounds or recognizing speech in ideal listening situations. Since they appear to "hear normally," the difficulties these individuals experience are often presumed to be the result of an attention deficit, a behavior problem, a lack of motivation, or some other cause. If this occurs, the individual may receive medical and/or remedial services that do not address the underlying "auditory" problem.

Central auditory processes are the auditory system mechanisms and processes responsible for the following behavioral phenomena:
- Sound localization and lateralization.
- Auditory discrimination.

- Temporal aspects of audition including: temporal resolution, temporal masking, temporal integration, and temporal ordering.
- Auditory performance with competing acoustic signals.
- Auditory performance with degraded signals.

These mechanisms and processes apply to nonverbal as well as verbal signals and may affect many areas of function, including speech and language (ASHA, 1996, p. 41).

What is Meant by the term "Central Auditory Processing?"
Katz, Stecker & Henderson (1992) described central auditory processing as "what we do with what we hear." In other words, it is the ability of the brain (i.e., the central nervous system) to process incoming auditory signals. The brain identifies sounds by analyzing their distinguishing physical characteristics frequency, intensity, and temporal features. These are features that we perceive as pitch, loudness, and duration. Once the brain has completed its analysis of the physical characteristics of the incoming sound or message, it then constructs an "image" of the signal from these component parts for comparison with stored "images." If a match occurs, we can then understand what is being said or we can recognize sounds that have important meanings in our lives (sirens, doorbells, crying, etc.).

This explanation is an oversimplification of the complicated and multifaceted processes that occur within the brain. The complexity of this processing, however, can be appreciated if one considers the definition of central auditory processing offered by the American Speech-Language-Hearing Association (ASHA).

This definition acknowledges that many neurocognitive functions are involved in the processing of auditory information. Some are specific to the processing of acoustic signals, while others are more global in nature and not necessarily unique to processing of auditory information (e.g., attention, memory, language representation). However, these latter functions are considered components of auditory processing when they are involved in the processing of auditory information.

What is Central Auditory Processing Disorder (CAPD)?
CAPD can be defined as a deficiency in any one or more of the behavioral phenomena listed above. There is no one cause of CAPD. In many children, it is related to maturational delays in the development of the important auditory centers within the brain. Often, these children's processing abilities develop as they mature. In other children, the deficits are related to benign differences in the way the brain develops. These usually represent more static types of problems (i.e., they are more likely to persist throughout the individual's life). In other children, the CAPD can be attributed to frank neurological problems or disease processes. These can be caused by trauma, tumors, degenerative disorders, viral infections, surgical compromise, lead poisoning, lack of oxygen, auditory deprivation, and so forth.

The prevalence of CAPD in children is estimated to be between 2 and 3% (Chermak & Musiek, 1997), with it being twice as prevalent in males. It often co-exists with other disabilities. These include speech and language disorders or delays, learning disabilities or dyslexia, attention deficit disorders with or without hyperactivity, and social and/or emotional problems.

What are some behavioral manifestations of CAPD?
Below is a listing of some of the common behavioral characteristics often noted in children with CAPD. It should be noted that many of these behavioral characteristics are not unique to CAPD. Some may also be noted in individuals with other types of deficits or disorders, such as attention deficits, hearing loss, behavioral problems, and learning difficulties or dyslexia. Therefore, one should not necessarily assume that the presence of any one or more of these behaviors indicates that the child has a CAPD. However, if any of these behaviors are noted, the child should be considered at risk for CAPD and referred for appropriate testing. Definitive diagnosis of a central auditory disorder cannot be made until specialized auditory testing is completed and other etiologies have been ruled out:

- Difficulty hearing in noisy situations.
- Difficulty following long conversations.
- Difficulty hearing conversations on the telephone.
- Difficulty learning a foreign language or challenging vocabulary words.
- Difficulty remembering spoken information (i.e., auditory memory deficits).
- Difficulty taking notes.
- Difficulty maintaining focus on an activity if other sounds are present child is easily distracted by other sounds in the environment.
- Difficulty with organizational skills.
- Difficulty following multi-step directions.
- Difficulty in directing, sustaining, or dividing attention.
- Difficulty with reading and/or spelling.
- Difficulty processing nonverbal information (e.g., lack of music appreciation).

There are a number of behavioral checklists that have been developed in an effort to systematically probe for behaviors that may suggest a CAPD (Fisher, 1976; Kelly, 1995; Smoski, Brunt, & Tannahill, 1992; Willeford & Burleigh, 1985). Some of these checklists were developed for teachers, while others were designed for parents. These checklists can be helpful in determining whether a child should be referred to an audiologist for a central auditory processing assessment.

Hearing Problems
Ask the following questions. If the answer is "yes" to three or more of these questions, the client may have a hearing problem and may need to have his/her hearing checked by a doctor.
- Do they have a problem hearing on the telephone?
- Do they have trouble hearing when there is noise in the background?
- Is it hard for them to follow a conversation when two or more people talk at once?
- Do they strain to understand a conversation?
- Do other people seem to mumble (or not speak clearly)?

- Do they misunderstand what others are saying and respond inappropriately?
- Do they often ask people to repeat themselves?
- Do they have trouble understanding the speech of women and children?
- Do others complain that the TV volume up too high?
- Do they hear a ringing, roaring, or hissing sound a lot?
- Do some sounds seem too loud?

What should you do?

Hearing problems are serious. The most important thing is to go see a doctor. The doctor may refer to an otolaryngologist (oh-toe-lair-in-GAH-luh-jist), a doctor who specializes in the ear, nose, and throat. An otolaryngologist will try to find out why the client has a hearing loss and offer treatment options. He or she may also refer to other hearing professionals, an audiologist (aw-dee-AH-luh-jist). An audiologist can measure hearing. Sometimes otolaryngologists and audiologists work together to find the right treatment. If a hearing aid is needed, an audiologist can help find the right one. Although children must be seen by a physician before they can be fitted for a hearing aid, adults do not always see a physician. Adults who do not see a physician before getting a hearing aid must sign a waiver.

Why do we lose hearing?

Hearing loss happens for many reasons. Some people lose their hearing slowly as they age. This condition is known as presbycusis (prez-buh-KYOO-sis). Doctors do not know why presbycusis happens, but it seems to run in families. Another reason for hearing loss may be exposure to too much loud noise. This condition is known as noise-induced hearing loss. Many construction workers, farmers, musicians, airport workers, tree cutters, and people in the armed forces have hearing problems because of too much exposure to loud noise. Sometimes loud noise can cause a ringing, hissing, or roaring sound in the ears, called tinnitus (tin-NY-tus).

Hearing loss can also be caused by a virus or bacteria, heart conditions or stroke, head injuries, tumors, and certain medicines.

What treatments and devices can help?

Treatment will depend on the hearing problem, so some treatments will work better than others. Here are the most common ones:

- **Hearing aids** are tiny instruments worn in or behind your ear. They make sounds louder. Things sound different when wearing a hearing aid, but an audiologist can help the client get used to it. To find the hearing aid that works best one may have to try several. Ask an audiologist for a trial period with a few different hearing aids. The audiologist can work together with the client until s/he is comfortable.

- **Personal listening systems** help hearing while eliminating or lowering other noises. Some, called auditory training systems and loop systems, make it easier to hear someone in a crowded room or group setting. Others, such as FM systems and personal amplifiers, are better for one-on-one conversations.

- **TV listening systems** help when listening to the television or the radio without being bothered by other noises. These systems can be used with or without hearing aids and do not require a very high volume.

- **Direct audio input hearing aids** are hearing aids that can be plugged into TVs, stereos, microphones, auditory trainers, and personal FM systems.

- **Telephone amplifying devices.** Some telephones are made to work with certain hearing aids. If a hearing aid has a "T" switch, ask your telephone company about getting a phone with an amplifying coil (T-coil). If the hearing aid is in the "T" position, this coil is activated when you pick up the phone. It provides a comfortable volume and helps lessen background noise. You can also buy a special type of telephone receiver and other devices to make sounds louder on the phone.

- **Mobile phone amplifying devices.** To help people who use a T-coil hear better on mobile phones, an amplifying device called a loopset is available. The wire loop goes around the neck and connects to the mobile phone. The loop transmits speech from the phone to the hearing aid. It also helps get rid of background noise to make it easier to talk in a noisy environment.

- **Auditorium-type assistive listening systems.** Many auditoriums, movie theaters, churches, synagogues, and other public places are equipped with special sound systems for people with hearing loss. These systems send sounds directly to the ears to help one hear better. Some can be used with a hearing aid and others without.
- **Cochlear** (COKE-lee-ur) **implants** have three parts: a headpiece, a speech processor, and a receiver. The headpiece includes a microphone and a transmitter. It is worn just behind the ear where it picks up sound and sends it to the speech processor, a beeper-sized device that can fit in your pocket or on a belt. The speech processor converts the sound into a special signal that is sent to the receiver. The receiver, a small round disc about the size of a quarter that a surgeon places under the skin behind one ear, sends a sound signal to the brain. Cochlear implants are most often used with young children born with hearing loss. However, older adults with profound or severe hearing loss are beginning to receive these implants more often.
- **Lip reading** or **speech reading** is another option. People who do this pay close attention to others when they talk. They watch how the mouth and the body move when someone is talking. Special trainers can help them learn how to lip read or speech read.

For more information, additional addresses and phone numbers, or a printed list of organizations, contact:

NIDCD Information Clearinghouse
1 Communication Avenue
Bethesda, MD 20892-3456
Toll-free Voice: (800) 241-1044
Toll-free TTY: (800) 241-1055
Fax: (301) 770-8977
E-mail: nidcdinfo@nidcd.nih.gov

Source: (Medline Plus)
Visual Problems
Definition
There are many types of eye problems and visual disturbances.
These include blurred vision, halos, blind spots, floaters, and other
symptoms. Blurred vision is the loss of sharpness of vision and the
inability to see small details. Blind spots (scotomas) are dark
"holes" in the visual field in which nothing can be seen. For the
most severe form of visual loss, see blindness.

Considerations
Changes in vision, blurriness, blind spots, halos around lights, or
dimness of vision should always be evaluated by a medical
professional. Such changes may represent an eye disease, aging,
eye injury, or a condition like diabetes that affects many organs in
your body.

Whatever the cause, vision changes should never be ignored. They
can get worse and significantly impact the quality of your life.
Professional help is always necessary. As you determine which
professional to see, the following descriptions may help:

- Opticians dispense glasses and do not diagnose eye
  problems.
- Optometrists perform eye exams and may diagnose eye
  problems. They prescribe glasses and contact lenses. In
  some states, they treat diseases that affect the eyes.
- Ophthalmologists are physicians who diagnose and treat
  diseases that affect the eyes. These doctors may also
  provide routine vision care services, such as prescribing
  glasses and contact lenses.

Sometimes an eye problem is part of a general health problem. In
these situations, your primary care provider should also be
involved.

Causes
Vision changes and problems can be caused by many different
conditions:

- Presbyopia -- difficulty focusing on objects that are close. Often becomes noticeable in your early to mid 40s.
- Cataracts -- cloudiness over the eye's lens, causing poor nighttime vision, halos around lights, and sensitivity to glare. Daytime vision is eventually affected. Common in the elderly.
- Glaucoma -- increased pressure in the eye, causing poor night vision, blind spots, and loss of vision to either side. A major cause of blindness. Glaucoma can happen gradually or suddenly -- if sudden, it's a medical emergency.
- Diabetic retinopathy -- this complication of diabetes can lead to bleeding into the retina. Another common cause of blindness.
- Macular degeneration -- loss of central vision, blurred vision (especially while reading), distorted vision (like seeing wavy lines), and colors appearing faded. The most common cause of blindness in people over age 60.
- Eye infection, inflammation, or injury.
- Floaters -- tiny particles drifting across the eye. Although often brief and harmless, they may be a sign of retinal detachment.
- Retinal detachment -- symptoms include floaters, flashes of light across your visual field, or a sensation of a shade or curtain hanging on one side of your visual field.
- Optic neuritis -- inflammation of the optic nerve from infection or multiple sclerosis. Clients may have pain when moving their eye or touch it through the eyelid.
- Stroke or TIA.
- Brain tumor.
- Bleeding into the eye.
- Temporal arteritis -- inflammation of an artery in the brain that supplies blood to the optic nerve.
- Migraine headaches -- spots of light, halos, or zigzag patterns are common symptoms prior to the start of the headache. An ophthalmic migraine is the visual symptoms without a headache.

Other potential causes of vision problems include fatigue, overexposure to the outdoors (temporary and reversible blurring of vision), and many medications.

Medications that can affect vision include antihistamines, anticholinergics, digitalis derivatives (temporary), some high blood pressure pills (guanethidine, reserpine, and thiazide diuretics), indomethacin, phenothiazines (like Compazine for nausea, Thorazine and Stelazine for schizophrenia), medications for malaria, ethambutol (for tuberculosis), and many others.

Home Care
Safety measures may be necessary if the client has vision problems. For example, if s/he has trouble seeing at night, they should not drive after dusk. It may be helpful to increase the amount of light in a room or arrange a home to remove hazards. A specialist at a low-vision clinic may be able to help.

When to contact a Medical Professional
Call a provider if:
- Trouble seeing objects to either side.
- Difficulty seeing at night or when reading.
- Gradual loss of the sharpness of your vision.
- Difficulty distinguishing colors.
- Blurred vision when trying to view objects near or far.
- Diabetes or family history of diabetes.
- Eye itching or discharge.
- Vision changes that seem related to medication (DO NOT stop or change a medication without talking to your doctor).

What to expect at an office Visit
The provider will check vision, eye movements, pupils, the back of the eye (called the retina), and eye pressure when needed. An overall medical evaluation will be done if necessary.

A Health provider will ask questions about vision problems, such as:

- When did this begin? Did it occur suddenly or gradually?
- How often does it occur? How long does it last?
- When does it occur? Evening? Morning?
- Is the problem in one eye or both eyes?
- Is vision blurred or is there double vision?
- Do you have blind spots?
- Are there areas that look black and missing?
- Is side (peripheral) vision missing?
- Are halos (circles of light) seen around shiny objects or lights?
- Do you see flashing lights or zigzag lines?
- Do you have sensitivity to light?
- Do stationary objects seem to be moving?
- Are colors missing? Is it difficult to differentiate colors?
- Is there pain?
- Are your eyes crossed? Does one or both of your eyes "drift"?
- Have you had an injury, infection, allergy symptoms, added stress or anxiety, feelings of depression, fatigue, or headache in the last few weeks to months? Have you been exposed to pollens, wind, sunlight, or chemicals in this time frame? Have you used any new soaps, lotions, or cosmetics?
- Is your vision better after you rest?
- Is it better with corrective lenses?
- Are there other symptoms present like redness, swelling, headache, pain, itching, discharge/drainage, a sense that something is in the eye, increased or decreased tearing, etc.?
- What medications do you take?
- Do you have diabetes or is there a family history of diabetes?

The following tests may be performed:
- Slit-lamp examination.

- Refraction test.
- Tonometry.

Treatments depend on the cause. Surgery will be recommended for some conditions (such as cataracts). Diabetics must control their blood-sugar level.

Prevention
Regular eye checkups from an ophthalmologist or optometrist are important. They should be done once a year if over age 65. A doctor will recommend earlier and more frequent exams if for clients with diabetes or who are already showing early signs of eye problems from diabetes, high blood pressure, or other causes.

The pressure in the eyes will be measured at some visits to test for glaucoma. Periodically, eyes will be dilated to examine the retina for any signs of problems from aging, high blood pressure, or diabetes.

These important steps can prevent eye and vision problems:
- Wear sunglasses to protect eyes.
- Don't smoke.
- Limit alcohol.
- Keep blood pressure and cholesterol under control.
- Keep blood sugars under control.
- Eat foods rich in antioxidants, like green leafy vegetables.

References
US Preventive Services Task Force. Screening for glaucoma: Recommendation statement. *Ann Fam Med.* 2005; 3(2): 171-172. Spierer A. Presbyopia among normal individuals. *Graefes Arch Clin Exp Ophthalmol.* 2003; 241(2): 101-105.

Source: (Maleskey)
Nutritional Deficiencies
Symptoms of Nutritional Deficiencies: What Your Doctor May Not See

Any of the following symptoms, and especially, if the client has several of them, it is time for a nutritional assessment.

1. Poor Night Time Vision

If they have trouble seeing in the dark or recovering nighttime vision after exposure to bright light, they may have a vitamin A and/or a zinc deficiency.

What to Take: Get vitamin A from orange-yellow foods and supplemental beta-carotene and mixed carotenoids, or from a multivitamin with a mix of both beta-carotene (2,500 IU) and preformed vitamin A (2,500 IU, but not more than 3,500 IU total). Get zinc from foods like seafood and meat and from a supplement containing at least 20 mg of zinc.

2. Muscle Pain and Weakness

If you've got more than your share, it's worth checking out two things: vitamin D deficiency, which has been linked to muscle pain and weakness and CoQ10, which can help to alleviate muscle pain and weakness caused by cholesterol-lowering statin drugs.

What to Take: Get at least 1,000-2,000 IU a day of vitamin D and 100-300 mg of CoQ10.

3. Depression

Even when you have good reasons to feel grumpy, your mood can be aggravated by poor diet. Good nutrition can also help antidepressant drugs work better.

What to Take: At least 1,00 IU of supplemental vitamin D, 500 mcg of vitamin B12 and 400-800 mcg of folic acid. Take 1,400 mg a day of fish oil.

4. Easy Bruising

People bruise more easily as they age, because they have less protective fat under their skin.

What to Take: Quercetin (600 mg) and vitamin C (500-1,000 mg a day) may help. Both improve capillary fragility. Vitamin K2 is also important. Get at least 100 mcg a day from leafy greens or a supplement. Other nutrients to take daily: copper (2 mg), zinc (20 mg), natural vitamin E (400 IU), vitamin B12 (500 mcg) and folic acid (400-800 mcg).

5. Tingly Feet and Wobbly Walking
Especially when it's accompanied by a loss of balance, tingly feet can be a sign of low vitamin B12. Low vitamin E or folic acid can also cause problems with the nerves in your feet.

What to Take: See your doctor for a complete work-up, and be sure to get at least 500 mcg of B12, 400-800 mcg of folic acid, and 400 IU of natural vitamin E every day.

6. Jumpiness
Both magnesium and thiamine deficiencies can cause an exaggerated sensitivity to noise, called a pronounced startle response. People who abuse alcohol are most likely to be deficient.

What to Take: At least 300-500 mg of magnesium and 50 mg of thiamine a day.

7. Burning Mouth
Symptoms may come and go, and include numbness and tingling.

What to Take: Get your iron levels checked. Take extra iron as recommended by your doctor. Take a multivitamin with at least 500 mcg of B12 and 400-800 mcg of folic acid.

8. Cracks in the Corners of Your Mouth
The medical term is angular cheilitis. These cracks look like paper cuts and are just as painful. They can lead to fungal, yeast or bacterial infection.

What to Take: A multivitamin with all eight B vitamins: thiamine (25 mg), riboflavin (25 mg), niacin (25 mg), vitamin B6 (50 mg), folic acid (400-800 mcg), B12 (500 mcg), biotin (300 mcg) and pantothenic acid (50 mg).

9. Bad Hair Every Day
Thinning, dry, brittle hair can be your cue to tune into your diet.

What to Take: 3-6 g of flax seed oil a day, plus a multi that has at least 300 mcg of biotin. Getting enough protein is important too.

10. Fragile Fingernails
White spots on nails can signal zinc deficiency. Spoon-shaped nails (they bend backwards) can mean low iron. Brittle, splitting nails can mean low calcium, zinc or a fatty acid deficiency.

Remedy: Get check for an iron deficiency and use supplemental iron as needed. Get 20 mg of zinc and 800-1,000 mg of calcium, and 6 g of flax seed oil a day.

11. Frequent Infections
We are all bombarded by germs, but people who are well-nourished do a better job of fending them off, because their immune systems have the resources they need to fight back.

What to Take: A multivitamin containing at least 500 mg of vitamin C and 20 mg of zinc, along with 1,000-2,000 IU of vitamin D.

The Anti-Aging Bottom Line: Nutritional deficiencies can seriously compromise your wellbeing and set the stage for many diseases. While symptoms can have many causes, poor nutrition is a cause that is often overlooked and easily corrected with the right supplements and better eating habits. Tune in with your body and take charge of your health so that you can live the longest, healthiest life possible.

Neurological Conditions

- Primary Neurodegenerative Disease
  - Diffuse Lewy Body Dementia
    - Note relation to Parkinson's disease, symptoms
    - Hallucinations, fluctuating course, neuroleptic hypersensitivity)
  - Fronto-temporal dementia
    - Impaired attention, behavioral dyscontrol
    - Decrease blood flow, hypometaboism on SPECT / PET
    - (Pick's disease, Argyrophylic grain disease)

Source: (National Institute of Neurological Disorders and Stroke)

Dementia with Lewy Bodies

Background

Frederick Lewy first described Lewy bodies (LBs), cytoplasmic inclusions found in cells of the substantia nigra in patients with idiopathic Parkinson's disease, in 1914. In the 1960s, several pathologists described patients with dementia who had LBs of the neocortex. However, such cases were presumed to be rare until the mid 1980s, when sensitive immunocytochemical methods to identify LBs were developed. Dementia with LBs (DLB) was then recognized as being far more common than previously thought.

The relationship of DLB and Parkinson's disease is an area of considerable controversy, particularly because dementia frequently occurs in Parkinson's disease. Many investigators believe that a spectrum of LB disorders exists.

The third report of the DLB Consortium headed by Ian McKeith discusses an arbitrary 1-year rule to distinguish DLB from Parkinson's disease with dementia.1 If parkinsonism has been present for 12 months or longer before cognitive impairment is detected, the disorder is called Parkinson's disease with dementia; otherwise, it is called DLB. The report recognizes that this rule may be difficult to apply in clinical practice. When dementia precedes motor signs, particularly with visual hallucinations and episodes of reduced responsiveness, the diagnosis of DLB should be considered. Clinical criteria for DLB were first proposed in 19962 and modified in the subsequent DLB Consortium reports3. Several clinicopathological studies have assessed the sensitivity and specificity of these clinical criteria.4, 5 These clinical features are discussed below.

Postmortem examinations in both Parkinson's disease and DLB patients demonstrate LBs in the substantia nigra and possibly in the locus ceruleus, dorsal raphe, substantia innominata, and dorsal motor nucleus of the vagus. LBs are found in the neocortex of many patients with idiopathic Parkinson's disease and in all patients with DLB. DLB overlaps parkinsonian dementias.

Pathophysiology
Symptoms and signs of DLB probably result, in part, from disruption of bidirectional information flow from the striatum to the neocortex, especially the frontal lobe. The cause is multifactorial. Altered neuromodulator and/or neurotransmitter levels (e.g., acetylcholine [ACh], dopamine) influence the function of many neuronal circuits. In DLB, nonpyramidal cells in layers V and VI of the neocortex may contain LBs. Their function in neocortical information processing and in relaying data to subcortical regions probably is impaired. The etiology of the fluctuations in cognitive function, which characterize DLB, is unknown.

Frequency
   United States
   Findings from autopsy studies suggest that DLB accounts for 10-20% of dementias. Up to 40% of patients with Alzheimer's disease have concomitant LBs. These mixed cases are sometimes called the LB variant of Alzheimer's disease (LBV-AD) and represent an overlap syndrome between DLB and Alzheimer's disease. Signs and symptoms of LBV-AD also overlap between DLB and Alzheimer's disease. Because the sensitivity and specificity

of clinical diagnosis are poor, no good epidemiologic data on incidence or prevalence of DLB are available.

International
Autopsy studies in Europe and Japan indicate that the frequency of DLB is comparable with that reported in studies from the United States.

Mortality/Morbidity
- Dementing illnesses (including DLB) shorten life expectancy.
- With severe disease, patients may experience swallowing problems that can lead to impaired nutrition.
- Patients are at risk for falls because of impaired mobility and balance.
- Because of prolonged bed rest, patients are at risk for decubitus ulcers.
- Dysphagia and immobility also can lead to pneumonia.

Physical
Patients usually have impaired cognition consistent with dementia. An important observation during mental status testing is that the client has periods of being alert, coherent, and oriented that alternate with periods of being confused and unresponsive to questions (although awake). This fluctuation is a relatively specific feature of DLB.
- Retrieval from memory may be relatively worse than memory storage.
- Patients may do relatively well with confrontation naming tests and poorly on tests of visuospatial skills (e.g., drawing a clock, copying figures).
- Patients may have some parkinsonian signs but usually not enough to meet the criteria for a diagnosis of Parkinson's disease.
- Mild gait impairment is relatively frequent and should not be ascribed to old age or osteoarthritis.
- Resting tremor occurs less frequently than in Parkinson's disease.

- Myoclonus may occur before severe dementia.

Causes
- The etiology of DLB is not known.
- Rare cases of familial DLB have been reported.
- Apolipoprotein E subtype 4 (ApoE4) genotype is overrepresented only when DLB occurs with concomitant Alzheimer's disease.

Medical Care
- Double-blinded, placebo-controlled studies have demonstrated that rivastigmine may decrease psychiatric symptoms associated with dementia with Lewy bodies (DLB), particularly apathy, anxiety, hallucinations, and delusions. These studies also demonstrate that patients with DLB treated with cholinesterase inhibitors do better on neuropsychological tests than subjects treated with placebo. Open-label studies suggest that donepezil and galantamine also are effective.
- For the treatment of agitation and hallucinations associated with DLB, acetylcholinesterase inhibitors should be tried first in most instances.
- In a small minority of patients, motor features are worsened with cholinesterase inhibitors.
- Levodopa/carbidopa may improve motor function in some patients with DLB; however, in many patients this combination has no effect and may exacerbate psychiatric symptoms or confusion.
- Hallucinations and agitation are especially troublesome in DLB. When these symptoms are mild, no medical treatment may be necessary.
- Acetylcholinesterase inhibitors should usually be tried first.
- Most experts recommend atypical neuroleptics such as clozapine, quetiapine, or aripiprazole when cholinesterase inhibitors are ineffective.
- Avoid standard neuroleptics such as haloperidol because of neuroleptic sensitivity.

- Depression is frequent in DLB patients and may result from damage in the dorsal raphe and locus ceruleus and/or as a psychological response to impaired function. Selective serotonin reuptake inhibitors are the drugs of choice.
- A few case reports have reported exacerbation of fluctuations with memantine.
- Some experts try antiepileptic drugs to treat agitation and hallucinations, but clinical data supporting their use is lacking.

Consultations

Spouses, family members, and caregivers of patients with DLB frequently realize that the client with DLB behaves differently than typical patients with Alzheimer's disease. Primary caregivers (or neurologists not specializing in dementia) frequently are unable to adequately explain these differences. In such situations, referral to a dementia specialist can be helpful.

Diet

No dietary restrictions are indicated except for patients with severe disease who have swallowing impairment.

Activity

Physical therapy and exercise classes can be useful to maintain mobility. Additionally, advise families of potential problems faced by patients with DLB who drive.

Source: (Mayo Clinic)

Frontotemporal Dementia

Definition

Frontotemporal dementia (frontotemporal lobar degeneration) is an umbrella term for a diverse group of uncommon disorders that primarily affect the frontal and temporal lobes of the brain — the areas generally associated with personality, behavior, and language.

In frontotemporal dementia, portions of these lobes atrophy, or shrink. Signs and symptoms vary, depending upon the portion of the brain affected. Some people with frontotemporal dementia undergo dramatic changes in their personality and become socially inappropriate, impulsive or emotionally blunted, while others lose the ability to use and understand language.

Frontotemporal dementia is often misdiagnosed as a psychiatric problem or as Alzheimer's disease. But frontotemporal dementia tends to occur at a younger age than does Alzheimer's disease, typically between the ages of 40 and 70.

Symptoms

Identifying precisely which diseases fall into the category of frontotemporal dementia presents a particular challenge to scientists. The signs and symptoms may vary greatly from one individual to the next. Researchers have identified several clusters of symptoms that tend to occur together and be dominant in subgroups of people with the disorder. More than one symptom cluster may be apparent in the same person.

Behavioral Changes

The most common signs and symptoms of frontotemporal dementia involve extreme changes in behavior and personality. These include:
- Increasingly inappropriate actions.
- Euphoria.
- Lack of judgment and inhibition.
- Apathy.
- Repetitive compulsive behavior.
- Decline in personal hygiene.
- Lack of awareness of thinking or behavioral changes.

Speech and Language Problems

Some subtypes of frontotemporal dementia are marked by the impairment or loss of speech and linguistic abilities. For example, primary progressive aphasia is characterized by an increasing difficulty in using and understanding written and spoken language.

People with another subtype, semantic dementia, utter grammatically correct speech that has no relevance to the conversation at hand.

Movement Disorders
Rarer subtypes of frontotemporal dementia are characterized by problems with movement, similar to those associated with Parkinson's disease or amyotrophic lateral sclerosis (ALS) — which is also often called Lou Gehrig's disease.

Movement-related signs and symptoms may include:
- Tremor.
- Rigidity.
- Muscle spasms.
- Poor coordination.
- Difficulty swallowing.
- Muscle weakness.

Lifestyle and Home Remedies
In some cases, caregivers can reduce behavior problems by changing the way they interact with people who have dementia. Examples include:
- Avoiding events or activities that trigger the behavior.
- Anticipating needs and alleviating them promptly.
- Maintaining a calm environment.

Coping and Support
Caring for someone with frontotemporal dementia is challenging and stressful because of the extreme personality changes and behavioral problems that frequently develop. Caregivers need assistance — from family members and friends, support groups, or respite care provided by adult care centers or home health care agencies.

When a person with frontotemporal dementia requires 24-hour care, most families turn to nursing homes. Plans made ahead of time will make this transition easier and may allow the person to be involved in the decision-making process.

Other Neurologic Conditions

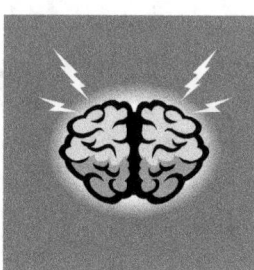

– Subdural hematoma
– Huntington's disease
– Creutzfeldt-Jakob disease
– Multiple sclerosis
– Corticobasal degeneration
– Cerebellar degeneration
– Progressive supranuclear palsy

Source: (Medical Dictionary)
Subdural Hematoma
Definition of Hematoma
Hematoma is a localized collection of blood, usually clotted, in a tissue or organ.

Description of Hematoma
Hematomas can occur almost anywhere on the body. In minor injuries, the blood is absorbed unless infection develops. Contusions (bruises) and black eyes are familiar forms of hematoma.

Less serious types include subungual hematoma (under a fingernail or toenail); hematoma auris (in the tissues of the outer ear, better known as cauliflower ear); and perianal hematoma (under the skin around the anus).

Hematomas are almost always present with a fracture. They are especially serious when they occur inside the skull, where they may place local pressure on the brain, notably epidural and subdural hematomas.

Treatment of Hematoma

Hematomas that occur intracranially require immediate specialized medical attention. For contusions (bruises), treatment consists of initially applying ice or cold packs a few times a day, to produce vasoconstriction (a reduction in arterial blood flow) which helps to decrease hemorrhage (bleeding) and edema (swelling). In general, the quicker you apply ice after the injury, the less bleeding will result.

If possible, elevate the bruised limb. Blood will leave the area of the wound and there may be less swelling. Resting the limb will also help to prevent further injury.

If the area is still painful after about 48 hours, apply gentle heat with warm towels, a hot water bottle, or a heating pad. The heat is applied for 20 minutes at a time to promote absorption and repair. Since heat causes swelling and increases tissue fluid, which may impair function, hot compresses may be followed by cold applications to minimize the secondary effects of heat.

Pressure in the form of an elastic adhesive bandage may be helpful to reduce hemorrhage and swelling. If infection should develop in the wound, the signs and symptoms might be increasingly severe pain, a fever of 101 degrees or more, swelling with surrounding redness, and pus. If any of these signs appear, your physician should be notified to make sure there are no additional problems.

Questions To Ask a Doctor About Hematoma
- What type of hematoma is this?
- What treatment is indicated?
- Will surgery be needed?
- Is complete recovery likely?

Source: (National Institute of Neurological Disorders and Stroke)

Huntington's Disease

What is Huntington's Disease?

Huntington's disease (HD) results from genetically programmed degeneration of brain cells, called neurons, in certain areas of the brain. This degeneration causes uncontrolled movements, loss of intellectual faculties, and emotional disturbance. HD is a familial disease, passed from parent to child through a mutation in the normal gene. Each child of an HD parent has a 50-50 chance of inheriting the HD gene. If a child does not inherit the HD gene, he or she will not develop the disease and cannot pass it to subsequent generations.

A person who inherits the HD gene will sooner or later develop the disease. Whether one child inherits the gene has no bearing on whether others will or will not inherit the gene. Some early symptoms of HD are mood swings, depression, irritability, or trouble driving, learning new things, remembering a fact, or making a decision. As the disease progresses, concentration on intellectual tasks becomes increasingly difficult and the client may have difficulty feeding himself or herself and swallowing.

The rate of disease progression and the age of onset vary from person to person. A genetic test, coupled with a complete medical history and neurological and laboratory tests, helps physicians diagnose HD. Presymptomic testing is available for individuals who are at risk for carrying the HD gene. In 1 to 3 percent of individuals with HD, no family history of HD can be found.

Is there any treatment?
Physicians prescribe a number of medications to help control emotional and movement problems associated with HD. In August 2008 the U.S. Food and Drug Administration approved tetrabenazine to treat Huntington's chorea (the involuntary writhing movements), making it the first drug approved for use in the United States to treat the disease. Most drugs used to treat the symptoms of HD have side effects such as fatigue, restlessness, or hyperexcitability. It is extremely important for people with HD to maintain physical fitness as much as possible, as individuals who exercise and keep active tend to do better than those who do not.

What is the prognosis?
At this time, there is no way to stop or reverse the course of HD. Now that the HD gene has been located, investigators are

continuing to study the HD gene with an eye toward understanding how it causes disease in the human body.

Source: (National Institute of Neurological Disorders)

Creutzfeldt-Jakob disease

What is Creutzfeldt-Jakob Disease?

Creutzfeldt-Jakob disease (CJD) is a rare, degenerative, invariably fatal brain disorder. Typically, onset of symptoms occurs at about age 60. There are three major categories of CJD: sporadic CJD, hereditary CJD, and acquired CJD. There is currently no single diagnostic test for CJD. The first concern is to rule out treatable forms of dementia such as encephalitis or chronic meningitis. The only way to confirm a diagnosis of CJD is by brain biopsy or autopsy. In a brain biopsy, a neurosurgeon removes a small piece of tissue from the client's brain so that it can be examined by a neurologist. Because a correct diagnosis of CJD does not help the client, a brain biopsy is discouraged unless it is need to rule out a treatable disorder. While CJD can be transmitted to other people, the risk of this happening is extremely small.

Is there any treatment?

There is no treatment that can cure or control CJD. Current treatment is aimed at alleviating symptoms and making the client as comfortable as possible. Opiate drugs can help relieve pain and the drugs clonazepam and sodium valproate may help relieve involuntary muscle jerks.

What is the prognosis?

About 90 percent of patients die within 1 year. In the early stages of disease, patients may have failing memory, behavioral changes, lack of coordination and visual disturbances. As the illness progresses, mental deterioration becomes pronounced and involuntary movements, blindness, weakness of extremities, and coma may occur.

Source: (Medline Plus)
Multiple Sclerosis (MS)
Multiple sclerosis (MS) is a nervous system disease that affects your brain and spinal cord. It damages the myelin sheath, the material that surrounds and protects your nerve cells. This damage slows down or blocks messages between your brain and your body, leading to the symptoms of MS. They can include:

- Visual disturbances.
- Muscle weakness.
- Trouble with coordination and balance.
- Sensations such as numbness, prickling, or "pins and needles."
- Thinking and memory problems.

No one knows what causes MS. It may be an autoimmune disease, which happens when your body attacks itself. Multiple sclerosis affects woman more than men. It often begins between the ages of 20 and 40. Usually, the disease is mild, but some people lose the ability to write, speak, or walk. There is no cure for MS, but medicines may slow it down and help control symptoms. Physical and occupational therapy may also help.

Treatments
Currently there is no cure for MS. However, there are treatments available that may slow
its progression and alleviate associated symptoms.

- **Drug therapies**—Medications that target the body's immune system may decrease the frequency and duration of attacks. These medications can be used on a long-term basis and also to treat specific attacks. Additional medications may be prescribed for other symptoms, such as pain or depression.

- **Additional therapies**—Because MS may affect the client's ability to perform self-care and other activities of daily living, treatment may also include referral to specialists for physical and occupational therapy.

Corticobasal Degeneration
What is Corticobasal Degeneration?
Corticobasal degeneration is a progressive neurological disorder characterized by nerve cell loss and *atrophy* (shrinkage) of multiple areas of the brain including the cerebral cortex and the basal ganglia. Corticobasal degeneration progresses gradually. Initial symptoms, which typically begin at or around age 60, may first appear on one side of the body (unilateral), but eventually affect both sides as the disease progresses. Symptoms are similar to those found in Parkinson disease, such as poor coordination, *akinesia* (an absence of movements), *rigidity* (a resistance to imposed movement), *disequilibrium* (impaired balance); and limb *dystonia* (abnormal muscle postures). Other symptoms such as cognitive and visual-spatial impairments, apraxia (loss of the ability to make familiar, purposeful movements), hesitant and halting speech, *myoclonus* (muscular jerks), and *dysphagia* (difficulty swallowing) may also occur. An individual with corticobasal degeneration eventually becomes unable to walk.

Is there any treatment?
There is no treatment available to slow the course of corticobasal degeneration, and the symptoms of the disease are generally resistant to therapy. Drugs used to treat Parkinson disease-type symptoms do not produce any significant or sustained improvement. Clonazepam may help the myoclonus. Occupational, physical, and speech therapy can help in managing disability.

What is the prognosis?
Corticobasal degeneration usually progresses slowly over the course of 6 to 8 years. Death is generally caused by pneumonia or other complications of severe debility such as sepsis or pulmonary embolism.

Source: (National Institute of Neurological Disorders and Stroke)
Cerebellar Degeneration
What is Cerebellar Degeneration?
Cerebellar degeneration is a disease process in which neurons in the cerebellum - the area of the brain that controls muscle coordination and balance - deteriorate and die. Diseases that cause cerebellar degeneration can also involve areas of the brain that connect the cerebellum to the spinal cord, such as the medulla oblongata, the cerebral cortex, and the brain stem. Cerebellar degeneration is most often the result of inherited genetic mutations that alter the normal production of specific proteins that are necessary for the survival of neurons.

Associated diseases: Diseases that are specific to the brain, as well as diseases that occur in other parts of the body, can cause neurons to die in the cerebellum. Neurological diseases that feature cerebellar degeneration include:

- **Acute and hemorrhagic stroke,** when there is lack of blood flow or oxygen to the cerebellum.
- **Cerebellar cortical atrophy, multisystem atrophy and olivopontocerebellar degeneration,** progressive degenerative disorders in which cerebellar degeneration is a key feature.
- **Friedreich's ataxia, and other spinocerebellar ataxias,** which are caused by inherited genetic mutations that progressively kill neurons in the cerebellum, brain stem, and spinal cord.
- **Transmissible spongiform encephalopathies** (such as "Mad Cow Disease" and Creutzfeldt-Jakob disease) in which abnormal proteins cause inflammation in the brain, particularly in the cerebellum.
- **Multiple sclerosis,** in which damage to the insulating membrane (myelin) that wraps around and protects nerve cells can involve the cerebellum.

Other diseases that can cause cerebellar degeneration include:
- **Endocrine diseases** that involve the thyroid or the pituitary gland.

- **Chronic alcohol abuse** that leads to temporary or permanent cerebellar damage.
- **Paraneoplastic disorders** in which tumors in other parts of the body produce substances that cause immune system cells to attack neurons in the cerebellum.

Symptoms: The most characteristic symptom of cerebellar degeneration is a wide-legged, unsteady, lurching walk, usually accompanied by a back and forth tremor in the trunk of the body. Other symptoms include slow, unsteady, and jerky movement of the arms or legs, slowed and slurred speech, and *nystagmus* -- rapid, small movements of the eyes.

Source: (National Institute of Neurological Disorders and Stroke)

Progressive Supranuclear Palsy

Progressive supranuclear palsy (PSP) is a rare brain disorder that causes serious and permanent problems with control of gait and balance. The most obvious sign of the disease is an inability to aim the eyes properly, which occurs because of lesions in the area of the brain that coordinates eye movements. Some patients describe this effect as a blurring. PSP patients often show alterations of mood and behavior, including depression and apathy as well as progressive mild dementia.

The disorder's long name indicates that the disease begins slowly and continues to get worse (*progressive*), and causes weakness (*palsy*) by damaging certain parts of the brain above pea-sized structures called nuclei that control eye movements (*supranuclear*).

PSP was first described as a distinct disorder in 1964, when three scientists published a paper that distinguished the condition from Parkinson's disease. It is sometimes referred to as Steele-Richardson-Olszewski syndrome, reflecting the combined names of the scientists who defined the disorder. Although PSP gets progressively worse, no one dies from PSP itself.

Who gets PSP?

Approximately 20,000 Americans - or one in every 100,000 people over the age of 60 - have PSP, making it much less common than Parkinson's disease, which affects more than 500,000 Americans. Patients are usually middle-aged or elderly and men are affected more often than women. PSP is often difficult to diagnose because its symptoms can be very much like those of other, more common movement disorders, and because some of the most characteristic symptoms may develop late or not at all.

What are the symptoms?

The most frequent first symptom of PSP is a loss of balance while walking. Patients may have unexplained falls or a stiffness and awkwardness in gait. Sometimes the falls are described by the person experiencing them as attacks of dizziness. This often prompts suspicion of an inner ear problem.

Other common early symptoms are changes in personality such as a loss of interest in ordinary pleasurable activities or increased irritability, cantankerousness, and forgetfulness. Patients may suddenly laugh or cry for no apparent reason, they may be apathetic, or they may have occasional angry outbursts, also for no apparent reason. It must be emphasized that the pattern of signs and symptoms can be quite different from person to person.

As the disease progresses, most patients will begin to develop a blurring of vision and problems controlling eye movement. In fact, eye problems usually offer the first definitive clue that PSP is the proper diagnosis. PSP patients have trouble voluntarily shifting their gaze downward, and also can have trouble controlling their eyelids. This can lead to involuntary closing of the eyes, prolonged or infrequent blinking, or difficulty in opening the eyes.

Another common visual problem is an inability to maintain eye contact during a conversation. This can give the mistaken impression that the client is hostile or uninterested.

Speech usually becomes slurred and swallowing solid foods or liquids can be difficult. In rare cases, some patients will notice shaking of the hands.

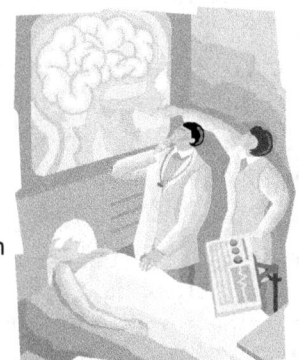

Trauma

- Concussion, Contusion
  - head trauma, if recent fall
- Subdural hematoma
- Hydrocephalus:
  - Normal pressure (late effect of bleed)
- Dementia pugilistica
- Possible contributor to Alzheimer's disease initiation and progression
- Concern: physical abuse by caretakers

Source: (Brain Injury.com)

Brain Trauma

Any brain function can be disrupted by brain trauma: excessive sleepiness, inattention, difficulty concentrating, impaired memory, faulty judgment, depression, irritability, emotional outbursts, disturbed sleep, diminished libido, difficulty switching between two tasks, and slowed thinking. Sorting out bonafide brain damage from the effects of migraine headaches, pain elsewhere in the body, medications, depression, preoccupation with financial loss, job status, loss of status in the community, loss of status in the family, and any ongoing litigation can be a formidable task.

The extent and the severity of cognitive neurologic dysfunction can be measured with the aid of neuropsychological testing. Neuropsychologists use their tests to localize dysfunction to specific areas of the brain. For example, the frontal lobes play an essential role in drive, mood, personality, judgment, interpersonal behavior, attention, foresight, and inhibition of inappropriate behavior. The ability to plan properly and execute those plans is known as "executive function." Frontal lobe injury is often associated with damage to the olfactory bulbs beneath the frontal lobes. Patients may note reduced or altered sense of smell. One recent study (Varney 1993) showed that 92% of brain injured client suffering anosmia (loss of smell) had ongoing problems with employment, even though their neuropsychological testing was relatively normal.

The effects of brain injury on the client may be equaled or even surpassed by the effect on the client's family. Brain injuries are known for causing extreme stressors in family and interpersonal relationships.

In general, symptoms of traumatic brain injury should lessen over time as the brain heals but sometimes the symptoms worsen because of the client's inability to adapt to the brain injury. For this and other reasons, it is not uncommon for psychological problems to arise and worsen after brain injury.

Symptom Checklist

A wide variety of symptoms can occur after "brain injury." The nature of the symptoms depends, in large part, on where the brain has been injured. Below find a list of possible physical and cognitive symptoms which can arise from damage to specific areas of the brain:

Frontal Lobe: forehead
- Loss of simple movement of various body parts (Paralysis).
- Inability to plan a sequence of complex movements needed to complete multi-stepped tasks, such as making coffee (Sequencing).
- Loss of spontaneity in interacting with others.
- Loss of flexibility in thinking.
- Persistence of a single thought (Perseveration).
- Inability to focus on task (Attending).
- Mood changes (Emotionally Labile).
- Changes in social behavior.

- Changes in personality.
- Difficulty with problem solving.
- Inability to express language (Broca's Aphasia).

Parietal Lobe: near the back and top of the head
- Inability to attend to more than one object at a time.
- Inability to name an object (Anomia).
- Inability to locate the words for writing (Agraphia).
- Problems with reading (Alexia).
- Difficulty with drawing objects.
- Difficulty in distinguishing left from right.
- Difficulty with doing mathematics (Dyscalculia).
- Lack of awareness of certain body parts and/or surrounding space (Apraxia) that leads to difficulties in self-care.
- Inability to focus visual attention.
- Difficulties with eye and hand coordination.

Occipital Lobes: most posterior, at the back of the head
- Defects in vision (Visual Field Cuts).
- Difficulty with locating objects in environment.
- Difficulty with identifying colors (Color Agnosia).
- Production of hallucinations.
- Visual illusions - inaccurately seeing objects.
- Word blindness - inability to recognize words.
- Difficulty in recognizing drawn objects.
- Inability to recognize the movement of object (Movement Agnosia).
- Difficulties with reading and writing.

Temporal Lobes: side of head above ears
- Difficulty in recognizing faces (Prosopagnosia).
- Difficulty in understanding spoken words (Wernicke's Aphasia).
- Disturbance with selective attention to what we see and hear.
- Difficulty with identification of, and verbalization about objects.

- Short term memory loss.
- Interference with long term memory.
- Increased and decreased interest in sexual behavior.
- Inability to categorize objects (Categorization).
- Right lobe damage can cause persistent talking.
- Increased aggressive behavior.

Brain Stem: deep within the brain
- Decreased vital capacity in breathing, important for speech.
- Swallowing food and water (Dysphagia).
- Difficulty with organization/perception of the environment.
- Problems with balance and movement.
- Dizziness and nausea (Vertigo).
- Sleeping difficulties (Insomnia, sleep apnea).

Cerebellum: base of the skull
- Loss of ability to coordinate fine movements.
- Loss of ability to walk.
- Inability to reach out and grab objects.
- Tremors.
- Dizziness (Vertigo).
- Slurred Speech (Scanning Speech).
- Inability to make rapid movements.

Amnesic Disorder
DSM-IV

A. Memory impairment
  - Inability to learn new information, or
  - Inability to recall previously learned information
- Memory disturbance significantly impairs social, occupational function, deterioration from past
- Memory not due to delirium, dementia
- Physiological basis or substance induced
  - Distinguish from dissociative disorders, dissociative amnesia, dissociative identity disorders
- Specify
  - Transient – less than 1 month
  - Chronic - more than 1 month

Source: (Wrong Diagnosis)

Amnesic Disorder

A partial or total loss of memory which can be caused by dementia, chronic alcohol abuse and nutritional deficiencies among others. Retrograde amnesia occurs when the person is unable to retrieve prior memories and antegrade amnesia is when a person is unable to form new memories.

How does aging change the brain?

When you're in your 20s, you begin to lose brain cells a few at a time. Your body also starts to make less of the chemicals your brain cells need to work. The older you are, the more these changes can affect your memory.

Aging may affect memory by changing the way the brain stores information and by making it harder to recall stored information.

Your short-term and remote memories aren't usually affected by aging. But your recent memory may be affected. For example, you may forget names of people you've met recently. These are normal changes.

Source: (Family Doctor)

Things to help memory:
- Keep lists.
- Follow a routine.
- Make associations (connect things in your mind), such as using landmarks to help you find places.
- Keep a detailed calendar.
- Put important items, such as your keys, in the same place every time.
- Repeat names when you meet new people.
- Do things that keep your mind and body busy.
- Run through the ABC's in your head to help you think of words you're having trouble remembering. "Hearing" the first letter of a word may jog your memory.

How does Alzheimer's disease change memory?
Alzheimer's disease starts by changing the recent memory. At first, a person with Alzheimer's disease will remember even small details of his or her distant past but not be able to remember recent events or conversations. Over time, the disease affects all parts of the memory.

How can I tell if memory problems are serious?
A memory problem is serious when it affects your daily living. If you sometimes forget names, you're probably okay. But you may have a more serious problem if you have trouble remembering how to do things you've done many times before, getting to a place you've been to often, or doing things that use steps, like following a recipe.

Another difference between normal memory problems and dementia is that normal memory loss doesn't get much worse over time. Dementia gets much worse over several months to several years.

It may be hard to figure out on your own if you have a serious problem. Talk to your family doctor about any concerns you have. Your doctor may be able to help you if your memory problems are caused by a medicine you're taking or by depression.

Memory problems that aren't part of normal aging:
- Forgetting things much more often than you used to.
- Forgetting how to do things you've done many times before.
- Trouble learning new things.
- Repeating phrases or stories in the same conversation.
- Trouble making choices or handling money.
- Not being able to keep track of what happens each day.

Source: (atHealth.com)

Dissociative Disorders
Symptoms
There are four major dissociative disorders:
- Dissociative amnesia.
- Dissociative identity disorder.
- Dissociative fugue.
- Depersonalization disorder.

Symptoms common to all types of dissociative disorders include:
- Memory loss (amnesia) of certain time periods, events and people.
- Mental health problems, including depression and anxiety.
- A sense of being detached from yourself (depersonalization) .
- A perception of the people and things around you as distorted and unreal (derealization).
- A blurred sense of identity.

Each of the four major dissociative disorders is characterized by a distinct mode of dissociation. Dissociative disorder symptoms may include:

Dissociative amnesia. Memory loss that's more extensive than normal forgetfulness and can't be explained by a physical or neurological condition is the hallmark of this condition. Sudden-onset amnesia following a traumatic event, such as a car accident, happens infrequently. More commonly, conscious recall of traumatic periods, events or people in your life — especially from childhood — is simply absent from your memory.

Dissociative identity disorder. This condition, formerly known as multiple personality disorder, is characterized by "switching" to alternate identities when you're under stress. In dissociative identity disorder, you may feel the presence of one or more other people talking or living inside your head. Each of these identities may have their own name, personal history, and characteristics, including marked differences in manner, voice, gender, and even such physical qualities as the need for corrective eyewear. There often is considerable variation in each alternate personality's familiarity with the others. People with dissociative identity disorder typically also have dissociative amnesia.

Dissociative fugue. People with this condition dissociate by putting real distance between themselves and their identity. For example, you may abruptly leave home or work and travel away, forgetting who you are and possibly adopting a new identity in a new location. People experiencing dissociative fugue typically retain all their faculties and may be very capable of blending in wherever they end up. A fugue episode may last only a few hours or, rarely, as long as many months. Dissociative fugue typically ends as abruptly as it begins. When it lifts, you may feel intensely disoriented, depressed, and angry, with no recollection of what happened during the fugue or how you arrived in such unfamiliar circumstances.

Depersonalization disorder. This disorder is characterized by a sudden sense of being outside yourself, observing your actions from a distance as though watching a movie. It may be accompanied by a perceived distortion of the size and shape of your body or of other people and objects around you. Time may seem to slow down, and the world may seem unreal. Symptoms may last only a few moments or may wax and wane over many years.

Treatments and Drugs

- **Psychotherapy** is the primary treatment for dissociative disorders. This form of therapy, also known as talk therapy, counseling or psychosocial therapy, involves talking about your disorder and related issues with a mental health professional. Your therapist will work to help you understand the cause of your condition and to form new ways of coping with stressful circumstances.

- **Psychotherapy** for dissociative disorders often involves techniques, such as hypnosis, that help you remember and work through the trauma that triggered your dissociative symptoms. The course of your psychotherapy may be long and painful, but this treatment approach often is very effective in treating dissociative disorders.

Source: (Mayo Clinic)

Other dissociative disorder treatments may include:

- **Creative art therapy.** This type of therapy uses the creative process to help people who might have difficulty expressing their thoughts and feelings. Creative arts can help you increase self-awareness, cope with symptoms and traumatic experiences, and foster positive changes. Creative art therapy includes art, dance and movement, drama, music and poetry.

- **Cognitive therapy.** This type of talk therapy helps you identify unhealthy, negative beliefs and behaviors and replace them with healthy, positive ones. It's based on the idea that your own thoughts — not other people or situations — determine how you behave. Even if an unwanted situation has not changed, you can change the way you think and behave in a positive way.

- **Medication.** Although there are no medications that specifically treat dissociative disorders, your doctor may prescribe antidepressants, anti-anxiety medications or tranquilizers to help control the mental health symptoms associated with dissociative disorders.

Causes of Amnesic Disorders

- Amnesia
  - Dissociative: localized, selective, generalized
  - Organic - damage to CA1 of hippocampus
    - thiamine deficiency (WKE), hypoglycemia, hypoxia
- Epileptic events
  - Partial complex seizures
- Specific brain diseases
  - Transient global amnesia
  - Multiple sclerosis

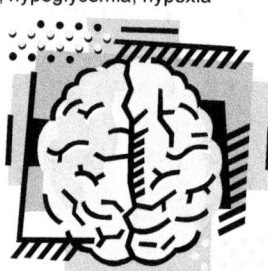

Source: (AtHealth)
What is amnesia?
Amnesia is a profound memory loss which is usually caused either by physical injury to the brain or by the ingestion of a toxic substance which affects the brain. In addition, the memory loss can be caused by a traumatic, emotional event.

What are the characteristics of amnesia?
People with amnesia have difficulty learning new information, and/or they have difficulty recalling previously learned information. They may be disoriented and confused. Their memory deficit causes problems for them either at work, in school, or in social settings. Sometimes the memory loss is severe enough to necessitate a supervised living situation.

Does amnesia affect males, females, or both?
Amnesia can affect anyone, male or female.

At what age does amnesia appear?
Amnesia can occur at any age.

How is amnesia diagnosed?
A mental health professional will want to take a careful personal history.

Causes of amnesia can include:
- External trauma, such as a blow to the head.
- Internal trauma, such as stroke.
- Exposure to a toxic substances such as carbon monoxide.
- Inadequate diet.
- Brain tumors.
- Seizures.

There are no laboratory tests that are necessary to confirm amnesia nor are there any physical conditions that must be met. However, it is very important not to overlook a physical illness that might mimic or contribute to amnesia. If there is any doubt about a medical problem, the mental health professional should refer to a physician, who will perform a complete physical examination and request any necessary laboratory tests.

Very sophisticated psychological testing, called neuropsychological testing, can be very helpful in determining the presence of amnesia. Sometimes the diagnosis of amnesia can be aided by the use of brain scans such as the magnetic resonance imaging (MRI).

How is amnesia treated?
Psychotherapy can be helpful for people whose amnesia is caused by emotional trauma. For instance, hypnosis may help some patients/clients recall forgotten memories.

Sometimes it is appropriate to administer a drug called Amytal (sodium amobarbital) to people suffering from amnesia. The medicine helps some people recall their lost memories. The use of hypnosis or Amytal has become controversial when it is used to help a client recall repressed memories, especially repressed memories associated with sexual abuse. After recalling memories of abuse, some patients have filed suit against the alleged perpetrator of the sexual abuse. The validity of memories recalled under these treatment situations is being questioned and tested in the courts.

Hospitalization is usually not necessary to treat amnesia unless the person is at risk for harming himself/herself.

What happens to people with amnesia?
The course of the amnesia is variable depending upon the cause of the memory problem. By removing the toxic substance, for instance alcohol, the person's memory will recover within hours. However, if the brain has been severely injured, it may take weeks, months, or years for recovery to occur. In some instances, the amnesia never goes away.

Therefore, the prognosis depends upon the extent of the brain trauma. If an ingested substance caused the memory loss and the body can rid itself of the offending substance without causing permanent brain injury, the prognosis is quite good. However, once the brain is damaged it may be very slow to heal, and therefore, the prognosis can be quite poor.

What can people do if they need help?
If you, a friend, or a family member would like more information and you have a therapist or a physician, please discuss your concerns with that person.

Source: (Merck)
Epileptic Events
Seizures
In seizure disorders, the brain's electrical activity is periodically disturbed, resulting in some degree of temporary brain dysfunction.

Many people have unusual sensations just before a seizure starts. Some seizures cause uncontrollable shaking and loss of consciousness, but more often, people simply stop moving or become unaware of what is happening.

Doctors suspect the diagnosis based on symptoms, but imaging of the brain, blood tests, and electroencephalography (to record the brain's electrical activity) are usually needed to identify the cause. If needed, drugs can usually prevent seizures.

Normal brain function requires an orderly, organized, coordinated discharge of electrical impulses. Electrical impulses enable the brain to communicate with the spinal cord, nerves, and muscles as well as within itself. Seizures may result when the brain's electrical activity is disrupted.

There are two basic types of seizures:
- **Epileptic:** These seizures have no apparent cause (or trigger) and occur repeatedly. These seizures are called a "seizure disorder" or "epilepsy."
- **Nonepileptic:** These seizures are triggered (provoked) by a disorder or another condition that irritates the brain. In children, a fever can trigger a nonepileptic seizure.

Certain mental disorders can cause symptoms that resemble seizures, called psychogenic nonepileptic seizures.

About 2% of adults have a seizure at some time during their life. Two thirds of these people never have another one. Most commonly, seizure disorders begin in early childhood or in late adulthood.

Causes
Causes are most common depend on when seizures start:

Before Age 2: High fevers or temporary metabolic abnormalities, such as abnormal blood levels of sugar (glucose), calcium, magnesium, vitamin B6, or sodium, can trigger one or more seizures. Seizures do not occur once the fever or abnormality resolves. If the seizures recur without such triggers, the cause is likely to be an injury during birth, a birth defect, or a hereditary metabolic abnormality or brain disorder.

2 to 14 Years: Often, the cause is unknown.

After Age 25: A head injury, stroke, or tumor may damage the brain, causing a seizure. Alcohol withdrawal (caused by suddenly stopping drinking) is a common cause of seizures. However, in about half of people in this age group, the cause is unknown.

Seizures with no identifiable cause are called idiopathic.

Conditions that irritate the brain—such as injuries, certain drugs, sleep deprivation, infections, fever—or that deprive the brain of oxygen or fuel—such as abnormal heart rhythms, a low level of oxygen in the blood, or a very low level of sugar in the blood—can trigger a single seizure whether a person has a seizure disorder or not. A single seizure that results from such a stimulus is called a provoked seizure (and thus is a nonepileptic seizure).

People with a seizure disorder are more likely to have a seizure when they are under excess physical or emotional stress or deprived of sleep. Avoiding these conditions can help prevent seizures. Rarely, seizures are triggered by repetitive sounds, flashing lights, video games, or even touching certain parts of the body. In such cases, the disorder is called reflex epilepsy.

Age-Associated Memory Impairment
vs
Mild Cognitive Impairment

- Memory declines with age
- Age - related memory decline corresponds with atrophy of hippocampus
- Older individuals remember more complex items and relationships
- Older individuals are slower to respond
- Memory problems predispose to development of Alzheimer's disease

Source: (NYU Medical Center)

Age Associated Memory Impairment A significant number of elderly individuals live with mild memory problems that are part of the normal aging process. Although many of these problems only mildly interfere with daily life, they may be troublesome to the person experiencing them.

Researchers have made progress in understanding the effects of aging on memory and continue to work toward treatments for age-associated memory problems.

Introduction
Age Associated Memory Impairment is a common condition characterized by very mild symptoms of cognitive decline that occur as part of the normal aging process. Symptoms confirmed in objective tests include a general slowness in processing, storing and recalling new information, and a general decline in the ability to perform tasks related to cognitive functioning (such as, memory, concentration, and organizing activities). Subjective complaints from individuals with age associated memory impairment often include difficulties remembering names and words. Current understanding of age associated memory impairment indicates that this condition is the result of physiological changes in the aging

brain and not a specific neurological disorder. Like every other organ of the body, the aging brain simply does not function quite as well as it used to.

Other designations for this condition include Age Related Cognitive Decline, Age Consistent Memory Impairment, and Late Life Forgetfulness.

Diagnosis

Age Associated Memory Impairment is a condition confirmed when diagnostic evaluation shows decline in cognitive abilities relative to former level of functioning that are not accompanied by evidence of neurological illness or other medical causes. Upon psychometric testing, cognitive performance is within the range of normal for age, and the cognitive decline has no significant impact on the ability to carry out everyday activities in the work or home setting. A diagnostic evaluation for Age Associated Memory Impairment includes neurological examinations, mental status examinations, neuropsychological and psychiatric evaluations, physical examination including laboratory tests, and a review of the client's past medical history and medications that the client is currently taking. An evaluation is complemented by clinical observations of the client's symptoms, their onset (sudden or gradual), presentation (how do symptoms occur), and progression of symptoms over time.

Progression

Symptoms of Age Associated Memory Impairment occur very gradually as a result of the normal aging process. Impairment may increase with age, but does not exceed a normal range of functioning for a particular age group.

Causes

Age Associated Memory Impairment is attributed to normal biological changes that occur as a person ages. In order to better understand this condition, researchers are studying these biological changes, as well as genetic and environmental factors that may have an impact on symptoms of Age Associated Memory Impairment.

Care and Treatment Options
Maintaining present health. Even when an evaluation shows that a person's symptoms are merely signs of Age Associated Memory Impairment and not a more serious memory problem, the person is still left with the difficulty of living with the potentially bothersome problem of forgetting. Although there are no treatments of proven value currently available for symptoms of Age Associated Memory Impairment, there are memory management strategies that may help a person overcome some of the symptoms.

Planning for the future. Although the memory problems a person may experience because of this condition do not indicate that a person will develop a more serious impairment, there is always a benefit to planning for one's future healthcare and long-term care. Planning ahead and putting one's wishes down in writing with documents such as healthcare proxies, living wills and powers of attorney for healthcare and finances are just some of the ways that one can plan for the future.

Why is an evaluation important for people with Age Associated Memory Impairment?
The symptoms of Age Associated Memory Impairment that a person may experience can cause unwarranted fear or anxiety that these may be early signs of Alzheimer's disease or another serious impairment. An evaluation serves to calm a person's fears, and provides an accurate picture of whether there are medical reasons causing the symptoms. Evaluations conducted every few years can help to monitor these symptoms over time.

Why is it important for clinicians and researchers to understand Age-Associated Memory Impairment?
Age Associated Memory Impairment can be troublesome to a person and affect his or her productivity and quality of life. Studying the causes and possible treatment of this condition may eventually lead to the reversal or prevention of the problem. Furthermore, in order to prevent or cure memory impairment or Alzheimer's disease, researchers and clinicians need to understand

which symptoms are indicators of disease and which are normal for a person at a certain age. Studying the symptoms of Age-Associated Memory Impairment is very important to this understanding because this condition marks the first stage in which individuals experience difficulties with memory. Also, it is important for researchers and clinicians to understand why some individuals experience only Age Associated Memory Impairment and why others develop Mild Cognitive Impairment or Alzheimer's disease.

Works Cited

Algiakrishnan, K. (n.d.). *Delirium*. Retrieved Nov 2010, from eMedicine: http://emedicine.medscape.com/article/288890-overview

atHealth. (n.d.). *Dissociative Disorders*. Retrieved Nov 2010, from Health - AtHealth.com: http://www.athealth.com/Consumer/disorders/Dissociative.html

AtHealth. (n.d.). *Dissociative Disorders*. Retrieved Nov 2010, from AtHealth.com: http://www.athealth.com/Consumer/disorders/Dissociative.html

Brain Injury.com. (n.d.). *Symptoms of Brain Injury*. Retrieved Nov 2010, from http://www.braininjury.com/symptoms.html

Depression guide. (n.d.). *Depression Definition*. Retrieved Nove 2010, from Depression-Guide.com: http://www.depression-guide.com/depression-definition.htm

eMedicine Health. (n.d.). *Depression*. Retrieved Sept 2010, from eMedicineHealth.com: http://www.emedicinehealth.com/depression/article_em.htm

Encyclopedia of Mental Disorder. (n.d.). *Delusions*. Retrieved Nov 2010, from Encyclopedia of Mental Disorder: http://www.minddisorders.com/Br-Del/Delusions.html

Encyclopedia of Mental Disorders. (n.d.). *Executive Function*. Retrieved Apr 2010, from Encyclopedia of Mental Disorders: http://www.minddisorders.com/Del-Fi/Executive-function.html

Family Doctor. (n.d.). *Memory Loss With Aging: What's Normal, What's Not*. Retrieved Nov 2010, from Family Doctor.org: http://familydoctor.org/online/famdocen/home/seniors/common-older/124.html

Health Central. (n.d.). *Agitation*. Retrieved Oct 2010, from HealthCentral.com: http://www.healthcentral.com/ency/408/003212.html

Help Guide.org. (n.d.). *Dealing with Depression: Self-Help and Coping Tips*. Retrieved Oct 2010, from HelpGuide.org: http://www.helpguide.org/mental/depression_tips.htm

Maleskey, G. (n.d.). *Symptoms of Nutritional Deficiencies: What Your Doctor May Not See*. Retrieved Nov 2010, from Live in the Now: http://www.stopagingnow.com/liveinthenow/article/symptoms-of-nutritional-deficiencies-what-your-doctor-may-not-see

Mayo Clinic. (n.d.). *Dissociative disorders*. Retrieved Nov 2010, from MayoClinic.com: http://www.mayoclinic.com/health/dissociative-disorders/DS00574/DSECTION=treatments-and-drugs

Mayo Clinic. (n.d.). *Early-onset Alzheimer's: When symptoms begin before 65*. Retrieved Oct 2010, from Mayo Clinic: http://www.mayoclinic.com/health/alzheimers/AZ00009

Mayo Clinic. (n.d.). *Frontotemporal Dementia*. Retrieved Sept 2010, from MayoClinic.com: http://www.mayoclinic.com/health/frontotemporal-dementia/DS00874

Medical Dictionary. (n.d.). *Hematoma*. Retrieved Nov 2010, from http://medical-dictionary.thefreedictionary.com/hematoma

Medline Plus. (n.d.). *Hallucinations*. Retrieved Apr 2010, from MedlinePlus: http://www.nlm.nih.gov/medlineplus/ency/article/003258.htm

Medline Plus. (n.d.). *Multiple Sclerosis*. Retrieved Oct 2010, from Medline Plus: http://www.nlm.nih.gov/medlineplus/multiplesclerosis.html

Medline Plus. (n.d.). *Vision Problems*. Retrieved Nov 2010, from Medline Plus: http://www.nlm.nih.gov/medlineplus/ency/article/003029.htm

Merck. (n.d.). *Agnosia*. Retrieved Nov 2010, from Merck Manuals Online Medical Library: http://www.merck.com/mmpe/sec16/ch210/ch210b.html

Merck. (n.d.). *Seizure Disorder*. Retrieved Nov 2010, from Merck: http://www.merck.com/mmhe/sec06/ch085/ch085a.html

National Institute of Deafness and Other Communication Disorders. (n.d.). *Apraxia of Speech*. Retrieved Nov 2010, from National Institutes of Health: http://www.nidcd.nih.gov/health/voice/apraxia.html

National Institute of Neurological Disorders . (n.d.). *NINDS Corticobasal Degeneration Information Page*. Retrieved Nov 2010, from NINDS: http://www.ninds.nih.gov/disorders/corticobasal_degeneration/corticobasal_degeneration.htm

National Institute of Neurological Disorders and Stroke. (n.d.). *NINDS Cerebellar Degeneration Information Page*. Retrieved Nov 2010, from NINDS: http://www.ninds.nih.gov/disorders/cerebellar_degeneration/cerebellar_degeneration.htm

National Institute of Neurological Disorders and Stroke. (n.d.). *NINDS Dementia With Lewy Bodies Information Page*. Retrieved Nov 2010, from National Institutes of Health: http://www.ninds.nih.gov/disorders/dementiawithlewybodies/dementiawithlewybodies.htm

National Institute of Neurological Disorders and Stroke. (n.d.). *NINDS Huntington's Disease Information Page*. Retrieved Nov 2010, from http://www.ninds.nih.gov/disorders/huntington/huntington.htm

National Institute of Neurological Disorders and Stroke. (n.d.). *NINDS Progressive Supranuclear Palsy Information Page*. Retrieved Nov 2010, from NINDS: http://www.ninds.nih.gov/disorders/psp/psp.htm

National Institute of Neurological Disorders. (n.d.). *Creutzfeldt-Jakob Disease Fact Sheet*. Retrieved Nov 2010, from http://www.ninds.nih.gov/disorders/cjd/detail_cjd.htm

NYU Medical Center. (n.d.). *Age Associated Memory Impairment*. Retrieved Nov 2010, from med.nyu.edu: http://www.med.nyu.edu/adc/forpatients/memory.html

Schminky, M. (1999). *Central Auditory Processing Disorders - An Overview of Assessment and Management Practices*. Retrieved Oct 2010, from exas School for the Blind and Visually Impaired: http://www.tsbvi.edu/seehear/spring00/centralauditory.htm

The Clements Clinic. (n.d.). *Treatment & Diagnosis*. Retrieved Nov 2010, from The Clements Clinic - A Healthy Change of Mind: http://www.clementsclinic.com/mood-disorders/treatments-diagnosis

The National Aphasia Association. (n.d.). *Aphasia Frequently Asked Questions*. Retrieved Nov 2010, from http://www.aphasia.org/Aphasia%20Facts/aphasia_faq.html

WebMD. (n.d.). *Depression and Diet*. Retrieved Nov 2010, from WebMD: http://www.webmd.com/depression/guide/diet-recovery

Wikipedia. (n.d.). *Disinhibition*. Retrieved Nov 2010, from http://en.wikipedia.org/wiki/Disinhibition

Wrong Diagnosis. (n.d.). *Amnesic Disorder*. Retrieved Nov 2010, from http://www.wrongdiagnosis.com/a/amnesic_disorder/intro.htm

Chapter 3 – Dementia Evaluations and Treatments

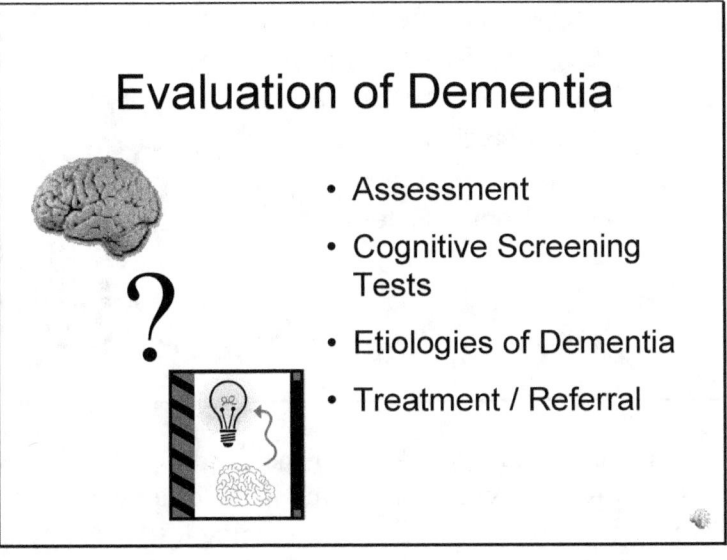

This chapter focuses on several aspects of the evaluation of dementia. First is discussed the general assessment of a demented client and cognitive screening tests that one might use. Next some of the specific etiologies of dementia, with a focus on the neurodegenerative varieties of dementia will be considered. Finally, treatment of the demented client and when to refer is noted.

Steps in Dementia Evaluation

- History
- Physical and Neurological Exam
- Cognitive Screening Test
- Rule out Reversible Causes
- Neuroimaging
- Consider Etiology
- Treatment or Referral

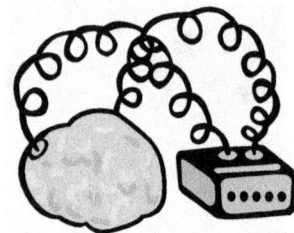

Above is shown the steps to take over the course of any dementia evaluation. This starts with history and includes a physical examination, a cognitive or memory screening test, some attempt to rule out potentially reversible causes of dementia and some type of brain scan.

Accuracy in diagnosis is an important part of the evaluation, and consideration of the cause of the dementia is important. Finally, with the advent of cognitive enhancers there are some compelling reasons to actively treat demented patients or at least to refer them for treatment.

History Taking

- Patient will "forget" their memory problems too
  - Get history from caregiver or spouse, if possible.

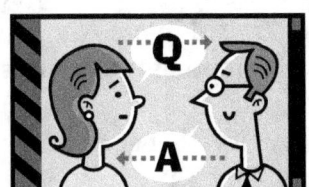

  - Memory impairment may be evidenced by repetitive questioning, list writing, lost objects, etc. .
  .

When it comes to evaluating a memory-impaired client, one must keep in mind that they will forget their own memory deficits. For this reason the most reliable history will come from a caregiver or spouse. Questions to ask about memory impairment in asking whether the client repetitively asks questions, writes lists, or loses objects.

History
The early diagnosis of dementia requires careful questioning to elicit clues to the presence of functional and cognitive impairment. Interviewing friends as well as family members is helpful, because family members may have adopted coping strategies to help the client with dementia, which sometimes conceal the client's impairment, making early diagnosis difficult. For example, a caregiver may take on additional responsibilities such as shopping and financial management, possibly masking the client's level of impairment.

During the medical history-taking, questions should be asked about forgetfulness and orientation. Inquiries should also be made regarding activities of daily living, including instrumental activities such as everyday problem solving and handling of business and financial affairs. Independent functioning in community affairs, such as job responsibilities, shopping, and participation in volunteer and social groups should be assessed. Evidence of problems with home activities, hobbies, and personal care should also be sought. In the early stages of dementia, the client may show restricted interest in hobbies and other activities, and may require prompting to maintain personal hygiene.

A variety of rating scales are available for evaluating cognitive function. Their use may or may not be required in the evaluation of early dementia.

Source: (National Library of Medicine, 1996)

Family History of Dementia

Data from family studies vary by type of dementia and are complicated by confounding variables. Evidence suggests that by age 90, about one-half of the first-degree relatives of dementia patients develop dementia (Breitner, Silverman, Mohs, et. al., 1988; Mohs, Breitner, Silverman, et. al., 1987). In their reanalysis of 11 case-control studies, van Duijn, Clayton, Chandra, et. al. (1991) reported an adjusted pooled odds ratio of 3.5 for family history. The risk is highest if a sibling was affected with Alzheimer's disease and increases with the number of first-degree relatives affected (Graves, White, Koepsell, et. al., 1990).

Genetic studies based on the evidence from family histories show that genetic factors contribute to the development of Alzheimer's disease. Autosomal-dominant forms of the disease typically appear at young ages and are usually associated with early death. At least three autosomal-dominant forms of the disease, all with early-onset symptoms, have been identified: a common one on chromosome 14 (Schellenberg, Bird, Wijsman, et. al., 1992; Sherrington, Rogaev, Liang, et. al., 1995) and rare ones on chromosome 1 (Levy-Lahad, Wijsman, Nemens, et. al., 1995) and chromosome 21.

It seems clear that other factors, such as other genes, life experiences, and environmental factors, must be involved to result in late-onset Alzheimer's disease. As Roses and colleagues (1994) suggest, it is not yet possible to depend on apoE genotyping for definitive guidance about diagnosis or treatment of Alzheimer's disease.

Instrumental Activities of Daily Living (IADL's)

- Telephone
- Travel
- Shopping
- Meals
- Housework
- Medicine
- Money

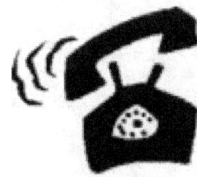
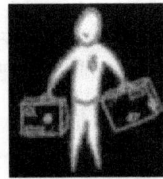
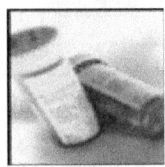
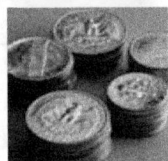

Once memory, is considered, next an examination about decline in functioning to meet diagnostic criteria is noted.

Source: (National Institute on Disabilities and Rehabilitation Research)
ADL's are "Activities of Daily Living." IADL's are the so-called "Instrumental Activities of Daily Living." the complexity of these activities is one step up from activities of daily living. It is useful to know whether the client's ability to perform these activities has declined in any way.

Instrumental Activities of Daily Living are usually listed as above, and include ability to use the telephone, to travel, to shop for one's self, to prepare meals, perform housework, take medications properly, and to handle money.

Activity	Need No Help (2 pts. each)	Need Some Help (1 pt. each)	Unable to Do At All (0 pts. each)
1. Using the Telephone	___	___	___
2. Getting to Places Beyond Walking Distance	___	___	___
3. Grocery Shopping	___	___	___
4. Preparing Meals	___	___	___
5. Doing Housework or Handyman Work	___	___	___
6. Doing Laundry	___	___	___
7. Taking Medications	___	___	___
8. Managing Money	___	___	___
Total Score			

Date: **Name:** **Activities of Daily Living**

Please check the box that most applies for each activity:

Source: (Lippincott's Nursing Center)

Instrumental Activities of Daily Living

Definition: Skills necessary to live independently, such as abilities to use a telephone, shop for groceries, handle finances, perform housekeeping tasks, prepare meals, and take medications.

The Lawton IADL scale takes 10 to 15 minutes to administer and contains eight items, with a summary score from 0 (low function) to 8 (high function). Each ability measured by the scale relies on either cognitive or physical function, though all require some degree of both. For example, a retrospective analysis by Cromwell and colleagues demonstrated an association between dependence in three items on the scale (using the telephone, self-medicating, and managing finances) and reduced cognitive function in community-dwelling older adults who hadn't been previously diagnosed with dementia. Low scores on other activities, such as housekeeping (a broad category encompassing simple tasks such as washing dishes or mowing the lawn), may more obviously point to problems in physical function.

The scale can be administered with a written questionnaire or by interview. The client or a knowledgeable family member or caregiver may provide answers. It is appropriate for use with older adults admitted to a hospital, a short-term skilled nursing facility, or a rehabilitation facility, as well as with community dwellers. The scale is generally not useful for older adults in long-term care facilities, where residents perform few IADLs without assistance.

Why Assess for Functional Decline?
Functional decline in older adults often begins within 48 hours of hospital admission and may lead to disability, institutionalization, and death. In a study of over 1,250 adults age 70 or older hospitalized for acute illness, Sager and colleagues found that 32% had declined in their ability to perform one or more ADLs by the time of discharge. After three months, 19% of participants reported the loss of an ADL, and 40% reported the loss of an IADL. Many factors contribute to immobility or inability to care for oneself during and after hospitalization:

- Physiologic and cognitive changes normal to aging.
- Disease or trauma such as pneumonia or hip fracture.
- Chronic conditions such as arthritis, diabetes, heart disease, or dementia.
- Cognitive impairment.
- Deconditioning resulting from reduced mobility.

Despite the Joint Commission's mandates for assessment of functional status upon admission and throughout the hospital stay, acute care hospitals use no standard criteria to identify patients at risk for functional decline. Functional assessment screening—using tools such as the Katz Index of Independence in Activities of Daily Living and the Lawton Instrumental Activities of Daily Living Scale—identifies a person's baseline functional status, including some components of mobility, such as the ability to transfer, and documents any changes that take place during hospitalization. Detailed knowledge of a client's strengths or deficits in self-care and mobility helps nurses plan appropriate rehabilitation both before and after discharge. Systematic functional assessment can also provide information on a client's response to treatments of acute illness or trauma.

Administering, Scoring, and Interpreting the Scale
Responses to each of the eight items in the scale will vary along a range of levels of competence—from independence in performing the activity to not performing it at all. It is not necessary to ask the questions in sequence as they appear on the tool. If a client is talking about shopping for groceries, it is fine to discuss transportation at that time as well. Or the interviewer may first ask, "What is your typical dinner?" before asking how the client prepares meals. If the client (or other informant) identifies independence with an activity, additional questions are unnecessary. If dependence in an activity is identified, additional information is needed to assess the extent of the deficit and how the deficit is accommodated.

In the late 1960s, Lawton and Brody used the scale to assess all eight domains of function for women but only five for men (food preparation, housekeeping, and laundry were excluded). While current practice is to include all eight domains for members of either sex, it may be useful to remember Ward and colleagues' observation that no IADL scale is right for every person, and "individualizing measures to only those activities which a person needs and wants to perform is a way of ensuring clinical relevance for individuals."

The Lawton IADL scale can be scored in several ways, depending on the goal of the assessment and how the information will be used. Vittengl and colleagues found that the scale had nearly equal validity in a population of rural older adults whether scored with simple or more complex systems. They concluded that, given time constraints, most clinicians will likely choose a faster, easier method of scoring. Based on my clinical experience and reading of the literature (which contains no systematic study of the relative frequency of the use of different scoring methods), the most common method is to rate each item either dichotomously (0 = less able, 1 = more able) or trichotomously (1 = unable, 2 = needs assistance, 3 = independent) and sum the eight responses. The higher the score, the greater the person's abilities.

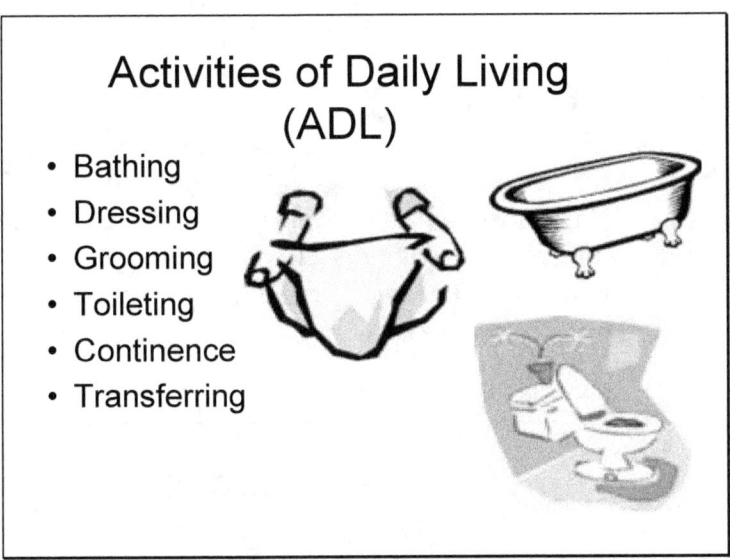

Activities of Daily Living (ADL)

- Bathing
- Dressing
- Grooming
- Toileting
- Continence
- Transferring

As the patients with dementia decline, they lose the ability to perform even rudimentary tasks. That is, they may be unable to perform even their ADL's or Activities of Daily Living. They may suffer from an inability to bathe, dress, and toilet or groom themselves. Incontinence can become a problem as can transferring from bed, chairs, or the toilet.

Date:_____ Name:_____ **Activities of Daily Living**

Function	Independent	Needs help	Dependent	Does Not do
Bathing				
Dressing				
Grooming				
Toileting				
Walking				
Climbing Stairs				
Eating				
Shopping				
Cooking				
Manage Medication				
Using the Phone				
Housework				
Doing Laundry				
Driving				

Source: (WebMD)

Activities of Daily Living (ADL)

Everyday routines generally involving functional mobility and personal care, such as bathing, dressing, toileting, and meal preparation. An inability to perform these renders one dependent on others, resulting in a self-care deficit. A major goal of occupational therapy is to enable the client to perform activities of daily living.

Importance of Cognitive Screening

- Establish a baseline level of functioning
- Allows for objective documentation of cognition
- Cognitive impairment is often not documented
  - Such patients are not evaluated for potentially reversible causes
  - They also do not receive treatment

Once history has been obtained and it seems that memory impairment and decreased level of functioning are both evident it is worth performing some type of brief cognitive screening test to establish a baseline and to have something objective to document.

Studies show that patients who are not documented to have memory deficits are not screened for potentially reversible causes. They also do not receive treatments specific to the memory deficits or to the behavioral problems associated with dementia.

Source: (UpToDate)
Cognitive Screening of Older Adults
The strongest risk factor for dementia is age, and the risk of dementia in the elderly increases with each decade. An estimated 11% of individuals 65 years of age and older, and 25-47% of individuals 85 years of age and older, have dementia.1 With the advent of pharmacological treatments for dementia, there is an increased need for cognitive screening of older adults. We will review indications to conduct cognitive screening in the elderly, cognitive screening instruments, and web resources for the newly diagnosed client.

The US Preventative Services Task Force (USPSTF) concluded there is insufficient evidence to recommend for or against routine screening for dementia in asymptomatic older adults. However, the USPSTF found "good evidence that some screening tests have good sensitivity but," unfortunately, "only fair specificity in detecting cognitive impairment and dementia." They concluded that there is "fair to good evidence that several drug therapies have a beneficial effect on cognitive function... but the evidence of their beneficial effects on instrumental activities of daily living is mixed, with the benefit being small at best.

The American Academy of Neurology and Canadian Task Force on Preventive Health Care reached similar conclusions. Further, a recent community-based study found that approximately half of the residents having independently in a retirement community were not willing to be screened routinely for memory problems. These results suggest that there is perceived harm associated with memory screening in asymptomatic individuals.

Dementia is a clinical diagnosis which relies upon an experienced clinician's assessment. Clinical methods for diagnosing dementia include assessing the presenting problem, obtaining focused history from a reliable informant, physical exam of the client, and evaluation of cognitive, behavioral, and functional status of the client. Given the time needed for mental status testing and clinical interview of client and informant, community physicians understandably fail to diagnosis dementia in over 50% of dementia cases, particularly in the earlier mild to moderate stages. By contrast, use of National Institute of Neurological and Communicative Disorder and Stroke and the Alzheimer's Disease and Related Disorders Association (NINCDADRDA)4 criteria by an experienced clinician for diagnosis of Alzheimer's disease can result in excellent diagnostic accuracy. Studies have found that from 85-93% of individuals diagnosed with AD in dementia specialty clinics have AD confirmed at autopsy.

Routine cognitive screening of all asymptomatic elderly may not be indicated, and this level of care would be costly and impractical. However, as noted by USPSTF, both the American Medical Association and American Academy of Family Physicians recommended that physicians be alert for cognitive and functional decline in elderly patients and for recognition of early stage dementia. Early recognition of cognitive impairment is important for multiple reasons including the high prevalence of mental status changes in the aged, diagnosis of potentially reversible medical conditions, initiation of treatment interventions, and to ensure that the client is able to adhere to medical recommendations. Early identification of cognitive decline gives patients and caregivers time to prepare for life style changes and plan for the future; e.g.;, arranging finances and discussing end-of-life care while the client is still competent.

Issues around driving an automobile provide a practical example of why early identification of dementia is important. Dementia is a major risk factor for unsafe driving and is associated with an increased rate of fatal accidents. Though specific cut off scores have not been established, impaired performance on brief cognitive screening tools such as the MMSE or clock drawing are related to impaired road test performance or caregiver report of hazardous driving. The presence of dementia does not necessarily preclude driving, but the majority of individuals with dementia will relinquish driving by three years after disease onset. Thus, early identification of dementia highlights the need to monitor key areas in an individual's life (financial management, driving) to prevent harm to self and others.

Issues around driving an automobile provide a practical example of why early identification of dementia is important. Dementia is a major risk factor for unsafe driving and is associated with an increased rate of fatal accidents. Though specific cut off scores have not been established, impaired performance on brief cognitive screening tools such as the MMSE or clock drawing are related to impaired road test performance or caregiver report of hazardous driving. The presence of dementia does not necessarily preclude driving, but the majority of individuals with dementia will relinquish driving by three years after disease onset. Thus, early identification of dementia highlights the need to monitor key areas in an individual's life (financial management, driving) to prevent harm to self and others.

The potential reversibility of some dementias has been a rationale for cognitive screening and a complete dementia work-up, which could include numerous costly tests, i.e. complete blood count, erythrocyte sedimentation rate, VDRL test for Syphilis, serum folate, serum cobalamin (B 12), chemistry panel, thyroid function studies, urinalysis, and brain imaging. Of note, the American Academy of Neurology abbreviated the list of recommended screening tests in the recent practice parameter. They recommended use of DSM-IV dementia criteria or the NINCDS-ADRDA diagnostic criteria, CT or MRI, screening for depression, B12 deficiency, and hypothyroidism. DSM-IV dementia criteria include impairment in memory, associated impairment in abstract thinking, impaired judgment, or other disturbances of higher cortical function or personality change, and gradual onset and continuing cognitive decline, severe enough to interfere significantly with work or usual social activities or relationships.

Numerous cognitive screening measures are available to assist in detection of dementia. An ideal screening instrument is standardized, reliable, and valid; has good sensitivity, specificity, positive and negative predictive value; and samples a range of cognitive functions. Ideally, scores should not be affected by changes related to normal aging, educational level, or race. The accuracy of screening tests for dementia has been reviewed and updated. The most widely used instrument in clinical practice is the Folstein Mini Mental Status Examination (MMSE). Its 30-point scale is heavily weighted with language and orientation items. It is most sensitive for Caucasian, high school educated individuals, with a generally recommended cut-off of 24/30, and 26/30 for college-educated individuals. Norms are available for diverse, less educated individuals, generally recommending a lower cut point (1 8/30). Positive predictive values range from 15-72% and negative predictive value from 95-99%' The Modified Mini Mental Status Examination (3MS) allows the clinician to obtain the traditional 30-point MMSE score as well as an expanded 1OO point score. A cutoff score of 86/100 has the best sensitivity but 77/100 has been used effectively in community-based screening (88% sensitivity, 90% specificity). The 3MS adds items typically impaired in Alzheimer's disease, such as category fluency and delayed recall memory.

Clock drawing test (CDT) (e.g. ask to draw a clock face, write all the numbers on the clock face and set the clock for 10 past 11), is a quick, simple measure, which can be scored reliably and encompasses multiple domains of cognition including executive and visuospatial functions. Using the CDT, dementia classification accuracy of 85% or more was found when normal older adults are compared to those with mild AD. Unfortunately, in very mild dementia, the CDT has poor sensitivity. The CDT is moderately to highly correlated with the MMSE and combined use of the CDT and MMSE increases detection of AD. The CDT was found to be more significantly related to driving impairment than the MMSE.

These are just a few of the Cognitive Screening tools available.

Screening Tests

- Mini-Mental State Exam (MMSE)
- Clock Drawing Test (CDT)
- Mini-Cognitive
- Time and Change
- 7-Minute Screen
- Others

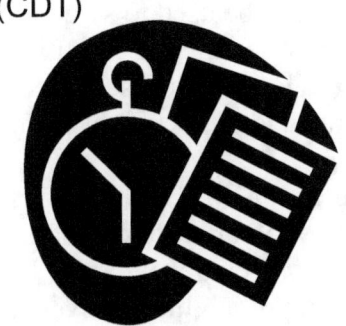

Mini-Mental Status Exam (MMSE)

- Orientation (10 points)
- Registration (3 points)
- Attention and Calculation (5 points)
- Recall (3 points)
- Language (8 points)
- Visuospatial (1 point)
- Total=30, if less than 25, consider dementia.

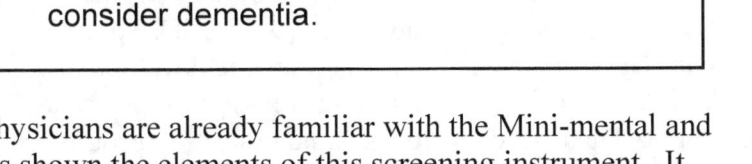

Most physicians are already familiar with the Mini-mental and above is shown the elements of this screening instrument. It covers several areas of cognition including memory, concentration, calculation, language, and visual-spatial abilities. The cutoff for dementia is generally held to be 25. However, there is a significant variation in scoring on this test based on age and education level.

Source: (QualityNet)
The MMSE is a brief, quantitative measure of cognitive status in adults. It can be used to screen for cognitive impairment, to estimate the severity of cognitive impairment at a given point in time, to follow the course of cognitive changes in an individual over time, and to document an individual's response to treatment.

The standard MMSE form published by PAR is based on its original 1975 conceptualization, with minor subsequent modifications by the authors. The MMSE has demonstrated validity and reliability in psychiatric, neurologic, geriatric, and other medical populations. The convenient new "all-in-one" test form includes a detachable sheet with stimuli for the Comprehension, Reading, Writing, and Drawing tasks. The form also includes alternative item substitutions for administration in special circumstances.

The pocket-size User's Guide provides detailed instructions for standard administration and scoring for each MMSE task, as well as recommended cutoff scores for use in classifying the severity of cognitive impairment. This handy pocket guide also provides population-based normative data (by age and years of education), which are useful for comparing an individual's MMSE Total score with the appropriate reference group, or when interpreting the scores of individuals who are illiterate, who have had less than 9 years of schooling, or who are 80 years of age or older.

MMSE Clinical Guide with Pocket Norms Card
The Clinical Guide by Marshal F. Folstein, MD, Susan E. Folstein, MD, and Gary Fanjiang, MD, describes the development, validation, administration, and interpretation of the MMSE. Normative data (*T* scores) for age and education groups are provided in the Appendix, as a supplement to the traditional interpretation of the MMSE raw scores.

Chapters in the Clinical Guide contain in-depth information about using the MMSE as part of the diagnostic process and highlight the instrument's usefulness in guiding psychiatric or medical treatment.

The MMSE test includes simple questions and problems in a number of areas: the time and place of the test, repeating lists of words, arithmetic, language use and comprehension, and basic motor skills. For example, one question asks to copy a drawing of two pentagons (shown on the right).

Interpretation
Any score over 27 (out of 30) is effectively normal. Below this, 20-26 indicates some cognitive impairment; 10-19 moderate to severe cognitive impairment, and below 10 very severe cognitive impairment. The normal value is also corrected for degree of schooling and age. Low to very low scores correlate closely with the presence of dementia, although other mental disorders can also lead to abnormal findings on MMSE testing. The presence of purely physical problems can also interfere with interpretation if not properly noted; for example, a client may be physically unable to hear or read instructions properly, or may have a motor deficit that affects writing and drawing skills.

Normative Data on MMSE

Education	Age (years)													
	18-24	25-29	30-34	35-39	40-44	45-49	50-54	55-59	60-64	65-69	70-74	75-79	80-84	>84
4th Grade	22	25	25	23	23	23	23	22	23	22	22	21	20	19
8th Grade	27	27	26	26	27	26	27	26	26	26	25	25	25	23
High School	29	29	29	28	28	28	28	28	28	28	27	27	25	26
College	29	29	29	29	29	29	29	29	29	29	28	28	27	27

Normative scores vary with age and education level!

This slide shows that there are normative scores available for the MMSE based on age and education level. For some people, then, 25 is clearly not the appropriate cutoff score. Rather it is the appropriate cutoff for an 80 year old with a high school education.

In other words, the score alone does NOT determine whether the individual meets criteria for the diagnosis or not.

```
┌─────────────────────────────────────────────────────────┐
│                                                         │
│            MMSE Pros and Cons                           │
│                                                         │
│   • Pros                                                │
│       – Widely used and therefore can track cognition   │
│         over time and between clinicians                │
│       – 5-10 minutes                                    │
│   • Cons                                                │
│       – False positives: those with little education    │
│       – False negatives: those with high premorbid      │
│         intellectual functioning                        │
│       – Psychologically stressful--makes people         │
│         angry                                           │
│                                                         │
└─────────────────────────────────────────────────────────┘
```

Pros and Cons

The most important advantage of the MMSE is that it is so widely used. It tends to be the standard score used by most clinicians and therefore can be used to track an individual client's cognitive abilities over time and between examiners. The test usually takes only 5-10 minutes. However, people with little education can show up as false positives on the test, and those with high intellect can show up as false negatives.

One disadvantage of the test is that it is psychologically stressful to take, and most people know that they are being tested. They can become quite anxious or even angry when asked the questions involved making the whole process quite unpleasant for everyone.

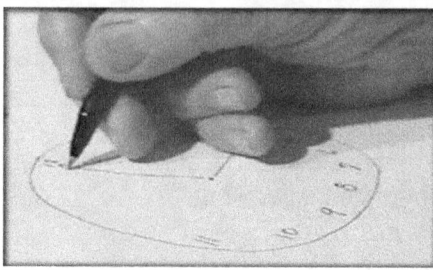

Clock Drawing Test (CDT)

- Draw a large circle on the (blank) page
- Put numbers on the circle
- Place hands to show 10 past 11
  - Tests planning, visuospatial abilities, but *not memory*
  - Less stressful, less culture-bound

An alternative to the Mini-Mental is the clock drawing test. I like this test because it is easy and short. It consists of merely asking the client to draw a large circle, preferably on a blank sheet of paper, put numbers on the circle to make it look like the face of a clock, and then to put hands on the clock to show that it is 10 past 11.

This does NOT test memory. However it does test planning, visuospatial abilities, and executive functioning. The most important thing is that it is relatively stress-free. The clock face is an image recognized across most cultures.

Source: (About.com: Alzeimer's Disease)
CDT
This is a simple test that can be used as a part of a neurological test or as a screening1 tool for Alzheimer's and other types of dementia.

The person undergoing testing is asked to:
- Draw a clock.
- Put in all the numbers.
- Set the hands at ten past eleven.

Scoring System for Clock Drawing Test (CDT)
There are a number of scoring systems for this test. The Alzheimer's disease cooperative scoring system is based on a score of five points.
- 1 point for the clock circle.
- 1 point for all the numbers being in the correct order.
- 1 point for the numbers being in the proper spaces.
- 1 point for the two hands of the clock.
- 1 point for the correct time.

A normal score is four or five points.

Test Results
The test can provide huge amounts of information about general cognitive and adaptive functioning such as memory, how people are able to process information and vision. A normal clock drawing almost always predicts that a person's cognitive abilities are within normal limits.

The Clock Drawing test does offer specific clues about the area of change or damage.
Research varies on the ability of the Clock Drawing test to differentiate between, for example, vascular dementia, and Alzheimer's disease. The CDT has been shown to lack sensitivity for mild cognitive impairment.

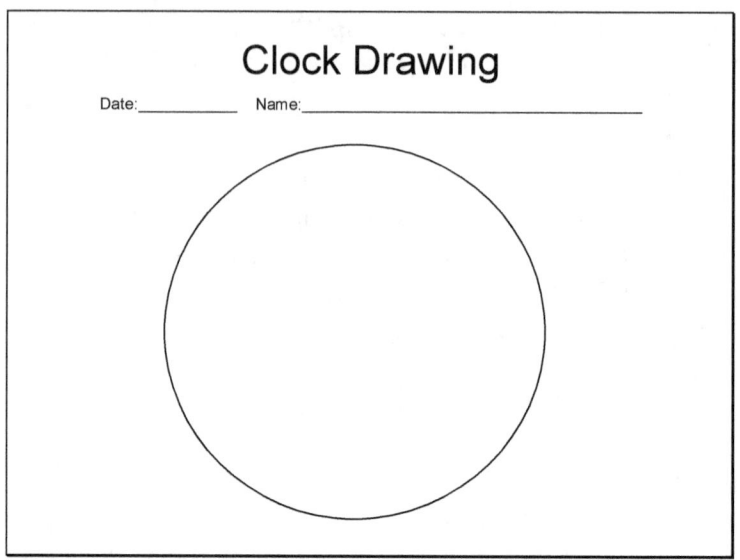

Be aware of lowing standards. Best practice includes developing very clear examples of what counts and what are out-side the norm. Evaluation drift is the tendency of the examiner to lower his/her standards as s/he administers an evaluation a number of times. Besides most of us want our clients to do well and find it difficult to come to terms with their declines.

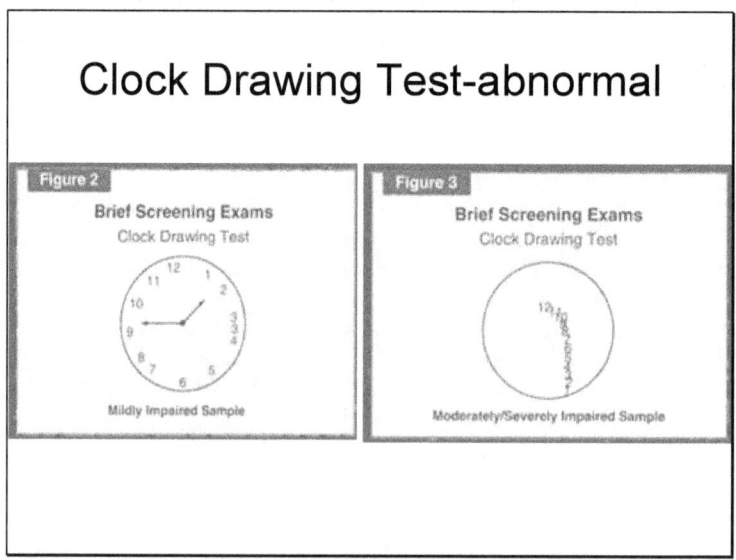

Here are a few examples of the Clock Drawing Test.

The clock on the left would be considered abnormal due the asymmetry of the digits on the clock.

The one on the right shows a more severe impairment.

Neither of these would be considered "normal"

Mini-Cognitive

- Clock-Drawing + three-item memory test
  - More sensitive than CDT
  - Same advantages as CDT
  - Not as commonly used
  - Involves visuospatial, executive and planning, and memory functions
- Concern = 2 word recall and/or abnormal clock

The "Mini-Cog" is simply the clock drawing test plus a three word memory test taken straight out of the Mini-Mental exam.

One would state three words; ask for understanding and hearing of the words; then do the CDT test; and then ask for the three words again.

An inability to remember at least 2 words and/or significant error on the clock drawing should indicate concern. This test is shorter than the MMSE and is quite sensitive.

Fast Diagnostic Test for Alzheimer's Disease and Dementia
  (1) First the client is asked to repeat three unrelated words. This is the same as in the Mini-Mental State Examination (MMSE).
  (2) The client is then asked to draw a clock. This is the same as the Clock Drawing Test (CDT).
  (3) The client is then asked to recall the three words.

Results of the Mini-Cog
If the client is unable to recall any of the three words then they are categorized as 'probably demented. If they can recall all three words then they are categorized as 'probably not demented'. People who can recall one or two words are categorized based on their clock drawing test.

Results of the Clock Drawing Test
If the client draws a clock that is in any way abnormal they are considered as 'probably demented'. If the clock is normally constructed then they are considered 'probably not demented'.

The Mini-Cog test results only contribute to a diagnosis of dementia. The test cannot be used in isolation in diagnostic tests for Alzheimer's disease.

Time and Change Test

- Telling Time Task: Patient asked to tell time when presented with clockface set at 11:10. Two tries allowed within 60 seconds.
- Making Change Task: Present patient with 3 quarters, 7 dimes, 7 nickels. Ask them to give one dollar's worth of change. Two tries within 120 seconds.

Technique: Time and Change Test
- Show client a clock face set to 11:10 and ask the time.
- Time the response and allow for up to one minute.
- Allow client 2 tries for a correct response.

Change making:
- Set client up with supply of loose change:
  - Quarters: 3.
  - Dimes: 7.
  - Nickels: 7.
- Ask client to put together one dollar in change.
- Time the response and allow up to two minutes.
- Better sensitivity if limit response to 12 seconds.
- Allow client 2 tries for a correct response.

Interpretation
Good: Correct response on both tests.
Concern: Incorrect response on either test.

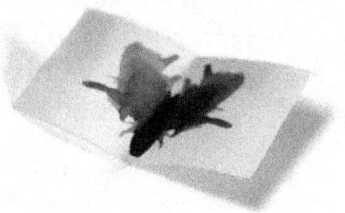
Many disorders resulting in dementia are partially or completely reversible, but in most studies these disorders account for less than 20 percent of patients with dementia.

Despite the relatively modest percentages represented by reversible causes of dementia, as well as treatable aspects of nonreversible dementias, it is important to recognize them. The potential to reverse the condition or halt or delay deterioration is among the most compelling justifications for early recognition of a dementing disorder. Knowledge of the client and alertness to changes suggesting dementia can trigger timely actions or referrals that enhance quality of life and, in the case of delirium, even save lives.

As noted, among the most frequent reversible causes of dementia are depression (depressive pseudodementia), alcohol abuse, and drug toxicity. Katzman, Lasker, and Bernstein (1988) reviewed diagnoses in nine published series of clinical cases and found that drug toxicity was the most common cause of reversible dementia (2.7 percent of all cases). Other causes of dementia, such as normal-pressure hydrocephalus, neoplasms, metabolic disorders, trauma, and infection, occurred less often.

Few studies of potentially reversible dementia have provided follow-up of identified cases to determine if the patients improved with treatment. Of the 32 studies analyzed by Clarfield (1988), had follow up. In the approximately 13 percent of patients with potentially reversible causes of dementia, only 11 percent actually improved with treatment, and only 3 percent had complete reversal.

Alcohol. Of the several toxins that can produce dementia, alcohol is associated with the highest frequency of dementia. The increasing incidence of alcoholism in older persons makes this an important consideration. Prolonged, heavy ingestion of alcohol may result in an amnestic disorder with cognitive deficits limited to memory impairment that is not a classic dementia by DSM-IV criteria (American Psychiatric Association, 1994;Brust, 1993;O'Brien, 1994;Victor, Adams, and Collins, 1989). This disorder, Wernicke-Korsakoff syndrome, is generally attributed to associated thiamine deficiency. Alcohol amnestic syndrome often follows an acute episode of Wernicke's encephalopathy; if the Wernicke's encephalopathy is treated early, alcohol amnestic syndrome could be prevented. Once this syndrome is established, there is generally only slight improvement over time.

A dementia that does meet DSM-IV criteria, alcohol-induced persisting dementia, has also been associated with prolonged, heavy ingestion of alcohol (American Psychiatric Association, 1994;Brust, 1993;O'Brien, 1994). This dementia persists after alcohol intake has stopped, and the etiologic role of alcohol in this disorder is controversial. Other nutritional disorders, such as multiple vitamin, protein, and calorie deficiencies, occur commonly in chronic alcoholics and have been linked to cognitive impairment. Correcting these deficiencies may improve cognitive function to some extent.

Drugs. Drug use, particularly drug interaction resulting from polypharmacy (the administration of many drugs together), is a common cause of cognitive decline in elderly persons. Physicians often prescribe agents such as antidepressants, antiarrhythmics, antihypertensives, analgesics, and derivatives of digitalis simultaneously, without attention to their effects on cognition. For some of these drugs, the effects can be additive or synergistic. Moreover, frequent use of hypnotic medication for sleep in elderly persons can lead to a constant state of confusion or delirium. Withdrawal of centrally acting agents, particularly antidepressants, hypnotics, and analgesics, can improve cognitive function significantly. Clinical experience also suggests that in older persons the "short-acting" psychotropic agents have longer-lasting effects. Clinicians should be alert to the signs of drug interactions. They can encourage the client and family members or caregivers to keep a complete record of all the client's medications, dosages, and schedules of administration, and to bring that record with them on each visit to a health care provider. A reminder that, for the purposes of recordkeeping, "medications" includes nonprescription products such as aspirin can be helpful. Patients may not know that most pharmacies will be pleased to keep a computerized record of medications prescribed by all their physicians.

Psychiatric Disorders. Clinically significant numbers of patients who present with apparent dementia have a major psychiatric disorder that accounts for their cognitive problems. Estimates range from 1 to 31 percent of persons diagnosed with progressive dementing illness. Depression is often misdiagnosed as dementia and vice versa. The AHCPR-sponsored guideline, *Depression in Primary Care: Volume 1. Detection and Diagnosis*, offers a detailed discussion of diagnosis and treatment of depression (Rush, Golden, Hall, et. al., 1993). Other psychiatric conditions that sometimes present with or mimic manifestations of dementia include schizophrenia (especially the paranoid form), bipolar disorders, and severe personality disorders. Given the frequency of a dementia misdiagnosis involving a psychiatric problem, follow-up monitoring, and continuity of care are especially valuable in ensuring that the client has been correctly diagnosed and is receiving suitable treatment. Indeed, the fact that psychiatric disorders can mimic dementia is one reason for undertaking the steps involved in initial assessment of an apparent dementing disorder.

Normal-Pressure Hydrocephalus. This is a disorder in which an abnormal accumulation of fluid in the cerebral ventricles compresses the brain. It is important as a diagnostic consideration because it is one of the causes of potentially reversible dementia. Although normal-pressure hydrocephalus is generally reported to account for less than 2 percent of all cases of dementia, some series indicate that it accounts for up to 6 percent of all cases. It occurs in middle-aged and older persons and is associated with dementia consisting of memory loss, confusion, slowness to respond, and paucity of thought that occurs over the course of weeks to years. Gait apraxia and urinary incontinence are also usually present. Although the condition may result from subarachnoid hemorrhage, trauma, or meningeal infection, most patients have no known precipitating illness or event.

Potentially Reversible Dementias

- Drug Toxicity
- Metabolic Disturbance
- Normal Pressure Hydrocephalus
- Mass Lesion (Tumor, Chronic Subdural)
- Infectious Process (Meningitis, Syphilis)
- Collagen-Vascular Disease (SLE, Sarcoid)
- Endocrine Disorder (Thyroid, Parathyroid)
- Nutritional Disease (B12, thiamine, folate)
- Other (COPD, CHF, Liver Disease, Apnea…)

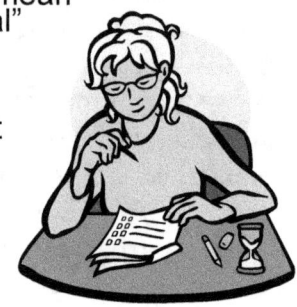

Potentially Reversible Causes

- Fewer than 13% reversible

  - Treatment does not mean they return to "normal"

  - "Treatable" a more appropriate term, but usually not "curable"

Most dementias are not reversible. In fact, fewer than 13% of all dementia cases may be "reversible." Furthermore, even when appropriate treatment is provided, most people do not return to normal or baseline cognitive functioning. Therefore, "treatable" is probably a more appropriate term than "reversible" or "curable."

Nonreversible Dementias
Alzheimer's disease and a small number of other disorders cause most cases of nonreversible dementia. More inclusive discussions of nonreversible dementias are available in articles by Katzman and Rowe (1992); Katzman, Terry, and Bick (1978); Khachaturian (1985); O'Brien (1994); Small and Jarvik (1982); Whitehouse (1993); and Wurtman, Corkin, Growdon, et. al. (1990). Nonreversible disorders aside from Alzheimer's disease are discussed below. Other relatively rare conditions also have nonreversible dementia as a feature.

Vascular Dementia. Vascular dementia, generally cited as the second most common of the nonreversible dementias, results from loss of neuronal tissue through death of brain tissue caused by interruption of blood supply, for example, by atherosclerotic lesions or from emboli. Hypertension with resultant cerebral infarctions is the most important, recognized, and preventable risk factor for vascular dementia; emboli from the heart or elsewhere within the vascular system are other causes. Vascular dementia frequently presents with a stepwise progression of symptoms, each with an abrupt onset, often in association with a neurologic incident. Focal neurologic findings, changes in tone and reflexes, and pseudobulbar palsy are common features of the illness. Vascular dementia is generally classified as a nonreversible dementia; however, appropriate treatment of hypertension and other risk factors for cerebrovascular disease is critical for prevention of further damage.

Pick's Disease. Pick's disease is a neurodegenerative disease characterized by severe cortical atrophy, most prominently of the frontal and temporal lobes. Persons with Pick's disease commonly show early signs of severe frontal lobe or temporal lobe dysfunction, characterized by general decline in mental function, changes in behavior patterns, and lack of insight. Later, loss of retentive memory, loss of language functions, and prominent grasp and sucking reflexes may occur. The disease is relentlessly progressive, generally over the course of 2 to 7 years, with the later stages characterized by features attributable to damage of the basal ganglia. The condition is usually sporadic but can occur in families.

Parkinson's Disease. Parkinson's disease is a progressive neurodegenerative disorder characterized by rigidity, bradykinesia, tremor, and postural instability resulting in disturbances of speech, gait, and coordination. Dementia associated with Parkinson's disease is insidious in onset and heralded by disorientation at night; its etiology has not been determined (Cedarbaum and Gancher, 1992;Yahr and Bergmann, 1986). Some cognitive impairment occurs in a large percentage of persons with Parkinson's disease; estimates range from 22 to 40 percent (Celesia and Wanamaker, 1972; Sroka, Elizan, Yahr, et. al., 1981). Overall, Parkinson's disease accounted for about 1 percent of all instances of dementia in the studies analyzed by Clarfield (1988) and in the neuropathologic series of Katzman and Rowe (1992).

AIDS-Related Dementia. Although AIDS-related dementia (also referred to as "AIDS-related complex") is uncommon in older persons, it warrants diagnostic consideration for patients with a suspected history of risk factors or behaviors, such as pre-1985 transfusions, history of unprotected sex, and injection drug use. As described in the DSM-IV (American Psychiatric Association, 1994), where it is called "dementia due to HIV disease," AIDS-related dementia is characterized by forgetfulness, slowness, poor concentration, and difficulties with problem solving. Prominent behavioral symptoms include apathy and social withdrawal. Physical examination may reveal tremor, impaired rapid repetitive movements, imbalance, ataxia, hypertonia, generalized hyperreflexia, positive frontal release signs, and impaired pursuit and saccadic eye movements (Arendt, Hefter, Neuen-Jacob, et. al., 1993;Kaeming and Kaszniak, 1989).

Neuroimaging

- Most treatment guidelines call for brain scan
  - CT usually adequate
  - MRI if Vascular Dementia suspected
  - "Small areas of white matter ischemic changes"--a common, seen in normals
  - Functional Imaging--not in initial workup

Some type of brain scan should also be included in a dementia workup. A CT is usually suffices to reveal any type of space-occupying lesion or normal pressure hydrocephalus. One might wish to consider an MRI particularly if vascular dementia is suspected or if there is some other type of structural abnormality that a CT might not pick up.

The finding of small areas of white matter ischemic change is common in this population of patients. This finding alone does not usually warrant a diagnosis of vascular dementia. In fact many people who are cognitively "normal" may have this finding. The question that arises though is whether or not they already have some type of neurodegenerative changes (i.e. early Alzheimer's) which finally comes to clinical attention only after these small vessel changes have occurred.

Finally, functional imaging, i.e. PET scanning is an increasingly inexpensive option. However, functional imaging usually is more helpful in differentiating between types of neurodegenerative dementias. These tests would be of limited value in the initial workup.

Establish Diagnosis

- Consider cause, because:
  - Treatments exist
  - Responses to treatments vary
  - Prognoses vary
  - Allows clinician to provide family with more meaningful information regarding the future

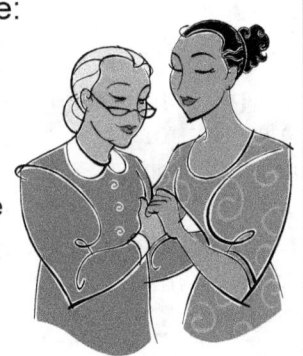

Now with some useful treatments for dementia, it makes more sense to come up with a working diagnosis than before. It is important that, although subtle, differences between the subtypes of dementia do exist. Therefore, the treatments for dementia can vary as can the responses to treatment.

Finally, prognoses are somewhat variable as well. Knowing the specific diagnosis of dementia allows the clinician to provide patients and families with more meaningful information regarding the disorder.

Even if the doctor diagnoses an irreversible form of dementia, much still can be done to treat the client and help the family cope. A person with dementia should be under a doctor's care, and may see a neurologist, psychiatrist, family doctor, internist, or geriatrician. The doctor can treat the client's physical and behavioral problems and answer the many questions that the person or family may have.

For some people in the early and middle stages of Alzheimer's disease, the drug Aricept is prescribed to possibly delay the worsening of some of the disease's symptoms. Doctors believe it is very important for people with multi-infarct dementia to try to prevent further strokes by controlling high blood pressure, monitoring and treating high blood cholesterol and diabetes, and not smoking.

Many people with dementia need no medication for behavioral problems. But for some people, doctors may prescribe medications to reduce agitation, anxiety, depression, or sleeping problems. These troublesome behaviors are common in people with dementia. Careful use of doctor-prescribed drugs may make some people with dementia more comfortable and make caring for them easier.

A healthy diet is important. Although no special diets or nutritional supplements have been found to prevent or reverse Alzheimer's disease or multi-infarct dementia, a balanced diet helps maintain overall good health. In cases of multi-infarct dementia, improving the diet may play a role in preventing more strokes.

Family members and friends can assist people with dementia in continuing their daily routines, physical activities, and social contacts. People with dementia should be kept up to date about the details of their lives, such as the time of day, where they live, and what is happening at home or in the world. Memory aids may help in the day-to-day living of patients in the earlier stages of dementia. Some families find that a big calendar, a list of daily plans, notes about simple safety measures, and written directions describing how to use common household items are very useful aids.

Source: (AtHealth)
Advice for Today
Scientists are working to develop new drugs that someday may slow, reverse, or prevent the damage caused by Alzheimer's disease and multi- infarct dementia. In the meantime, people who have no dementia symptoms can try to keep their memory sharp.

Some suggestions include developing interests or hobbies and staying involved in activities that stimulate both the mind and body. Giving careful attention to physical fitness and exercise also may go a long way toward keeping a healthy state of mind. Limiting the use of alcoholic beverages is important, because heavy drinking over time can cause permanent brain damage.

Many people find it useful to plan tasks; make "things-to-do" lists; and use notes, calendars, and other memory aids. They also may remember things better by mentally connecting them to other meaningful things, such as a familiar name, song, or lines from a poem.

Stress, anxiety, or depression can make a person more forgetful. Forgetfulness caused by these emotions usually is temporary and goes away when the feelings fade. However, if these feelings last for a long period of time, getting help from a professional is important. Treatment may include counseling or medication, or a combination of both.

Some physical and mental changes occur with age in healthy people. However, much pain and suffering can be avoided if older people, their families, and their doctors recognize dementia as a disease, not part of normal aging.

In some cases, appropriate treatment for the underlying condition can resolve dementia completely or partially. The type of treatment depends on the condition. For example, antibiotics are used to treat infection, and surgery is performed to remove a blood clot or tumor.

The goal of treatment for irreversible conditions is to control symptoms. Three FDA-approved drugs may provide symptomatic relief for Alzheimer's: donepezil (Aricept®), galantamine (Reminyl®), and rivastigmine (Exelon®).

Tranquilizers and sedatives can ease agitation, anxiety, and aggression. Medications or devices may be used to help manage sleeplessness and incontinence. Safety precautions are necessary to protect a person who is disoriented and may wander from home. Many patients with dementia eventually require 24-hour care in a health or residential facility.

Treatment

- Focus on behavior – not reason
  - Behavior = Communication

  - ABCs of behavior

  - Utilize strengths

  - Reward/recognize appropriate behavior

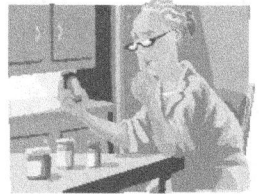

Source: (HealthLine)
Behavioral Therapy
Traditionally, behavioral therapy has been based on principles of

conditioning and learning theory using strategies aimed
at suppressing or eliminating challenging behaviors. More
recently, positive programming methodologies (La Vigna &
Donnellan, 1986) have used non-aversive methods in helping to
develop more functional behaviors. Moniz-Cook (1998) suggests
that behavioral analysis is often the starting point of most other
forms of therapeutic intervention in this area. Furthermore, she
suggests that modern behavioral approaches can be wholly
consistent with person-centered care. Behavioral therapy requires
a period of detailed assessment in which the triggers, behaviors
and reinforces (also known as the ABC: antecedents, behaviors and
consequences) are identified and their relationships made clear to
the client. The therapist will often use some kind of chart or diary
to gather information about the manifestations of a behavior and
the sequence of actions leading up to it. Interventions are then
based on an analysis of these findings. Emerson (1998) suggests
focusing on three key features when designing an intervention:
taking account of the individual's preferences; changing the
context in which the behavior takes place; and using reinforcement
strategies and schedules that reduce the behavior.

The efficacy of behavioral therapy has been demonstrated in the
context of dementia in only a small number of studies (Burgio &
Fisher, 2000).For example, there is evidence of
successful reductions in wandering, incontinence and other forms
of stereotypical behaviors (Woods, 1999).Meares & Draper
(1999) presented case studies testifying to the efficacy of
behavioral therapy, but they noted that the behaviors had diverse
causes and maintaining factors, and advised that behavioral
interventions must be tailored to individual cases.

Source: (Wikipedia)
Validation Therapy
Validation therapy was developed as an antidote to the
perceived lack of efficacy of reality orientation. It was suggested
by its originator, Naomi Feil, that some of the features
associated with dementia such as repetition and retreating into the
past were in fact active strategies on the part of the affected
individual to avoid stress, boredom and loneliness. She argues that

people with dementia can retreat into an inner reality based on feelings rather than intellect, as they find the present reality too painful.

Validation therapy therapists therefore attempt to communicate with individuals with dementia by empathizing with the feelings and meanings hidden behind their confused speech and behavior. It is the emotional content of what is being said that is more important than the person's orientation to the present. There have been relatively few empirical studies assessing the efficacy of the validation approach, as noted by Feil (1967), Mitchell (1987) and Hitch (1994). Hitch noted that validation therapy promotes contentment, results in less negative affect and behavioral disturbance, produces positive effects and provides the individual with insight into external reality. It was, however, suggested that therapists could become too focused on confused communication and could fail to identify simple explanations such as pain or hunger. Neal & Briggs (2002) evaluated validation therapy across a number of controlled trials, employing cognitive and behavioral measures. They concluded that despite some positive indicators, the jury was still out with respect to its efficacy.

Source: (Alzheimer's Disease: Cause, Symptoms, Treament)
Reminiscence Therapy
Reminiscence therapy involves helping a person with dementia to relive past experiences, especially those that might be positive and personally significant, for example family holidays and weddings. This therapy can be used with groups or with individuals. Group sessions tend to use activities such as art, music, and artifacts to provide stimulation. Reminiscence therapy is seen as a way of increasing levels of well-being and providing pleasure and cognitive stimulation. Few high-quality studies have been conducted in this area, and Spector et.
al (2002*b*) identified only two randomized controlled trials. From their limited data-set they concluded that there was little evidence of a significant impact of the approach O'Donovan (1993), however, stated that, although there is little indication of cognitive improvement, there is some evidence suggesting improvements in

behavior, well-being, social interaction, self-care and motivation (Gibson, 1994). It is also claimed that premorbid aspects of the person's personality may re-emerge during reminiscence work (Woods, 1999). The therapy also has a great deal of flexibility as it can be adapted to the individual. A person with severe dementia can still gain pleasure from listening to an old record, for instance.

Treatment

- Art and Creative Projects
  - Meaningful stimulation
  - Social interactions
  - Improved self-esteem
- Music
  - Reduction in agitation
  - Reduction in adverse behaviors
- Pets
- Touch

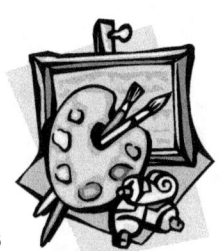

Source: (Healthy Woman)

Art Therapy

Art therapy has been recommended as a treatment for people with dementia as it has the potential to provide meaningful stimulation, improve social interaction, and improve levels of self-esteem (Killick & Allan 1999). Activities such as drawing and painting are thought to provide individuals with the opportunity for self-expression and the chance to exercise some choice in terms of the colors and themes of their creations.

Music Therapy

Several studies have reported benefits gained by people with dementia from music therapy (Killick & Allan, 1999). The therapy may involve engagement in a musical activity (e.g. singing or playing an instrument), or merely listening to songs or music. Lord & Garner (1993) showed increases in levels of well-being, better social interaction, and improvements in autobiographical memory in a group of nursing home residents who regularly had music played to them. Such improvements were not observed in a comparison group engaged in other activities. Cohen-Mansfield & Werner (1997) compared three types of intervention for people with abnormal vocalizations, and found that music therapy significantly reduced the behavior. More recently, a study by Gerdner (2000) found a significant reduction in agitation in people with dementia who were played an individualized program of music as opposed to traditional relaxation music.

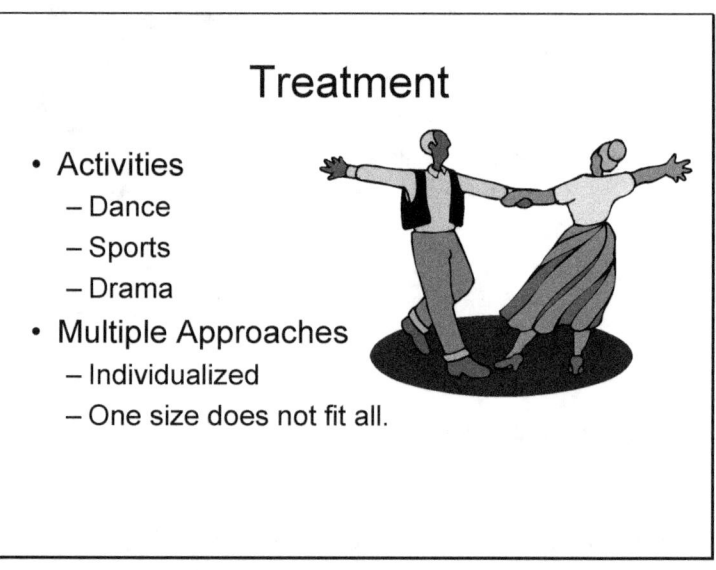

Source: (Douglas, 2004)

Activity Therapy

Activity therapy involves a rather amorphous group of recreations such as dance, sport and drama. It has been shown that physical exercise can have a number of health benefits for people with dementia, for example reducing the number of falls and improving mental health and sleep (King et. al, 1997) and improving their mood and confidence (Young & Dinan, 1994). In addition, Alessi et. al(1999) found in a small-scale controlled study that daytime exercise helped to reduce daytime agitation and nighttime restlessness. An interesting approach to dance therapy is described by Perrin (1998), who employed a form of dance known as 'jabadeo', which involves no prescriptive steps or motions but allows the participants to engage with each other in interactive movements. It is relevant to note that this may also fulfill a need for non-sexual physical contact which many people with dementia find soothing.

One striking thing is the move towards more person-centered forms of care (Kitwood, 1997). Within this approach, greater attempts are made to understand the individual's experience of dementia and to employ strategies to improve the person's quality of life. A further shared feature is the systemic perspective, that is, the need to work with systems (families, professional careers, organizations, etc.). Indeed, care staff and families are usually integral to treatment strategies. They are essential in obtaining valid and reliable information and constructing appropriate formulations. Also, there are keys to conducting any interventions reliably. It is evident, that training of careers (both professional and family) is an important part of most treatment programs. In fact, one study (Bird et. al, 2002) suggested that the most common interventions for psychological and behavioral symptoms of dementia were not necessarily specific therapies but working with careers or nursing home staff to change the attitudes and behavior of those in their care. Despite the relevance of this issue, there remain relatively few high-quality studies in the area (e.g. Marriott et. al, 2000). Clearly, training and support are important and worthy of further study; future studies need to be large and also include follow-up methodologies.

The field of dementia care is expanding, with an increasing number of articles on psychosocial interventions; to that extent the future looks promising. However, it is noted that there is a fundamental weakness within the current literature that clearly requires addressing. This concerns the limited attention paid to process issues (i.e. details outlining the mechanism of change underpinning the interventions). The available studies have been good at presenting the contents of intervention programs, but usually fail to outline how the interventions were conducted(communication strategies, interpersonal style, feedback mechanisms, staff training issues). Indeed, if these issues were better delineated, it would help therapists develop, refine, and improve the manner in which they implement their treatment programs (James et. al., 2003).

Treatment

- Some "Out of the Box" Suggestions
  - Message therapist
  - Audio books (Classics)
  - Audio journaling memoirs
  - Assign responsibilities
  - Recordings of old time radio shows
  - Old magazines
  - Music from their teenage/young adult years

Source: (LiveStrong)

Environmental Interventions and Dementia

Pleasurable mealtimes can enhance the quality of life of many nursing-home residents with dementia. Modifications in the environment can improve the dining experience, support the rehabilitation process, and enhance overall nutrition. The dining environment should ultimately help compensate for cognitive impairments, thus acting as a facilitator, and be easily modifiable to compensate for future impairments as residents' needs change. Assessing environmental stimuli, lighting, noise levels, staff care practices, and other aspects of the dining environment are not part of routine clinical practice for most speech-language pathologists. There are many situations in long-term care, however, in which residents with dementia who do not perform to their maximum potential or exhibit "behavior problems" may simply be responding to something in the environment that is not supportive.

The following environmental adjustments can make meals more enjoyable for residents.

Turn Up the Lights

Older individuals require three times the amount of light as younger individuals. Therefore, a dining room that is well-lit for residents may seem overly bright to younger caregivers. Corners are often not as well lit as other areas of the room. Try adding lights and directing the light so it bounces off the walls. Make sure not to point lights directly at shiny surfaces such as polished floors or tables, as older adult eyes are much less tolerant of glare than younger eyes.

Increase Visual Contrast

In addition to lighting, consider other aspects of the visual environment. Provide high contrast between the plate and the table or place setting. Research projects have shown that this change, along with increased light levels, can be effective in increasing independence and caloric intake (Brush, Threats, & Calkins, 2003; Koss & Gilmore, 1998; Brush, 2001). Also consider how the food is served. Some people will do better if they are given one course at a time. Too many choices may be overwhelming. Other research has shown an increase in intake with the use of primary-colored china (red or blue). This research suggests that nursing home staff and designers should consider modifying dining environment barriers, such as dim lighting and poor contrast, to increase clients' ability to participate in meals. These environmental changes—which support residents' independence—will facilitate favorable therapeutic outcomes.

Improve the Acoustics

Dining rooms seldom are carpeted, so it's important to look to other surfaces to absorb noise. If there are many windows (a hard surface that bounces noise instead of absorbing it), use full drapes or curtains around them to help absorb some noise. If the ceiling is high enough (usually 10 feet or more), fabric-covered acoustic panels that hang down several feet will both absorb noise and prevent reverberation. If ceiling panels are not feasible, add acoustic panels to the wall. Wood trim gives them an old-fashioned, elegant paneled effect.

Works Cited

About.com: Alzeimer's Disease. (n.d.). *Clock Drawing Test*. Retrieved Nov 2010, from http://alzheimers.about.com/od/diagnosisissues/a/clock_test.htm

Alzheimer's Disease: Cause, Symptoms, Treament. (n.d.). *Reminiscence Therapy for Alzheimers Treatment*. Retrieved Nov 2010, from http://alzheimers-review.blogspot.com/2010/06/reminiscence-therapy-for-alzheimers.html

AtHealth. (n.d.). *Forgetfulness:It's Not Always What You Think*. Retrieved Nov 2010, from http://www.athealth.com/consumer/disorders/forgetfulness.html

Douglas, S. (2004). Non-pharmacological Interventions in Dementia. *Advances in Psychiatric Treatment*, 171-179.

HealthLine. (n.d.). *Behavioral Therapy*. Retrieved Nov 2010, from HealthLine: http://www.healthline.com/galecontent/behavioral-therapy

Healthy Woman. (n.d.). *Music and Art Therapy as an Effective Treatment for People With Dementia*. Retrieved Oct 2010, from Article Alley: http://www.articlealley.com/article_1236810_17.html

Lippincott's Nursing Center. (n.d.). *The Lawton Instrumental Activities of Daily Living Scale*. Retrieved Nov 2010, from http://www.nursingcenter.com/library/JournalArticle.asp?Article_ID=781867

LiveStrong. (n.d.). *Environmental Interventions in Dementia*. Retrieved Nov 2010, from Livestrong.com: http://www.livestrong.com/article/109483-environmental-interventions-dementia/

National Institute on Disabilities and Rehabilitation Research. (n.d.). *Chartbook on Mental Health and Disability*. Retrieved Nov 2010, from http://www.infouse.com/disabilitydata/mentalhealth/appendices_glossary.php

National Library of Medicine. (1996, Nov). *Recognition and Initial Assessment of Alzheimer's Disease and Related Dementias*.

Retrieved Mar 2009, from National Library of Medicine:
http://www.ncbi.nlm.nih.gov/bookshelf/br.fcgi?book=hsarc
hive&part=A30948

QualityNet. (n.d.). *Mini-Mental Status Examination.* Retrieved
Nov 2010, from Qualitynet.com:
http://www.qualitynet.org/dcs/ContentServer?c=MQTools
&pagename=Medqic/MQTools/ToolTemplate&cid=11108
10465938

UpToDate. (n.d.). *Risk Factors for Dementia.* Retrieved Oct 2010,
from UpToDate.com:
http://www.uptodate.com/patients/content/topic.do?topicKe
y=~ZcncVEHyHWFMEw

WebMD. (n.d.). *activities of daily living.* Retrieved from
WebMD.com:
http://dictionary.webmd.com/terms/activities-of-daily-
living(adls)

Wikipedia. (n.d.). *Validation Therapy.* Retrieved Nov 2010, from
http://en.wikipedia.org/wiki/Validation_therapy

Chapter 4 - Alzheimer's Disease: Stages, Therapies, & Behaviors

It is important to compare dementia and Alzheimer's disease to realize the differences between the two conditions. Alzheimer's is the most common form of dementia marked by memory loss in older people. Dementia is the gradual loss of intellectual function. Alzheimer's statistics show that the disease can strike a person as early as 45, while dementia generally takes hold after age 70. The most confused form of dementia is Multi-Infarct Dementia or MID. This condition also attacks the blood vessels in the brain. Both disorders require testing to determine the best course of treatment.

Dementia and Alzheimer's diseases are perhaps two of the most confusing diseases that exist in the realm of mental degradation in America today. There are a number of differences, however, that allow for those dealing with symptoms characteristic of these two diseases to become more informed.

Comparing the Two Diseases
When comparing dementia vs. Alzheimer's disease it is very important to discuss the differences between the two diseases. Although they have many similarities, there are a number of differences that must be noted.

Alzheimer's disease is defined as a form of dementia characterized by the gradual loss of several important mental functions. It is perhaps the most common cause of dementia in older Americans, and goes beyond just normal forgetfulness, such as losing your car keys or forgetting where you parked. Signs of Alzheimer's disease include memory loss that is much more severe and more serious, such as forgetting the names of your children or perhaps where you have lived for the last decade or two.

Another way to compare dementia and Alzheimer's disease is to realize that dementia is a medical term used to describe a number of conditions characterized by the gradual loss of intellectual function. Certain symptoms, as defined by the American Medical Association, of dementia include memory impairment, increased language difficulties, decreased motor skills, failure to recognized or identify objects, and disturbance of the ability to plan or think abstractly.

Yet another way to determine the differences of dementia and Alzheimer's disease is when the onset of the disease was first noticed. Of course, this is a very difficult thing since the progression of both is very gradual, and often there is no one point where someone can say, "Aha!" and know that the disease has taken hold. Often the onset of Alzheimer's can occur as early as 45 years of age. General dementia, however, usually is noted later in life, perhaps in the 70 to 80 year range.

When looking at dementia and Alzheimer's disease, one type of dementia is often confused with Alzheimer's disease – Multi-Infarct Dementia or MID. MID is a common cause of dementia in the elderly and occurs when blood clots block small blood vessels in the brain and destroys brain tissue. Symptoms of MID, which are very similar to Alzheimer's disease, include confusion, problems with short term memory, wandering, and getting lost in familiar places, loss of bladder and bowel control, and emotional problems such as laughing or crying during inappropriate times.

Alzheimer's Disease

- Insidious onset and gradual progression

- Presentation usually related to primary deficits in recent memory

- Incidence age-related: 8%/year by 85

- 1/2-2/3 of time, cause of dementia is AD

- Ultimate diagnosis based on pathology of plaques and tangles

The first syndrome of dementia is also the most common, which is Alzheimer's. This form of dementia is characterized by a very insidious onset and a slow, gradual progression. The typical presentation of Alzheimer's involves a primary deficit in recent memory; behavioral problems; then executive problems tend to be noticed later. The incidence of dementia is age related. The incidence increases so that by the age of 85, there is an 8% incidence rate. As far as prevalence goes, 1/2-2/3 of all dementia cases are estimated to secondary to Alzheimer's disease.

Remember, though, the absolute diagnosis cannot be made until autopsy when extracellular plaques surrounding a beta-amyloid core are found throughout the cortex. Intracellularly, tangles are found within neurons that are composed of abnormally phosphorylated Tau proteins.

Alzheimer's Disease (AD)
Alzheimer's disease (AD) is the most common form of dementia among older people. Dementia is a brain disorder that seriously affects a person's ability to carry out daily activities.

AD begins slowly. It first involves the parts of the brain that control thought, memory, and language. People with AD may have trouble remembering things that happened recently or names of people they know. Over time, symptoms get worse. People may not recognize family members or have trouble speaking, reading or writing. They may forget how to brush their teeth or comb their hair. Later on, they may become anxious or aggressive, or wander away from home. Eventually, they need total care. This can cause great stress for family members who must care for them.

AD usually begins after age 60. The risk goes up as you get older. Your risk is also higher if a family member has had the disease. No treatment can stop the disease. However, some drugs may help keep symptoms from getting worse for a limited time.

In a very few families, people develop AD in their 30s, 40s, and 50s. This is known as "early onset" AD. These individuals have a mutation in one of three different inherited genes that causes the disease to begin at an earlier age. More than 90 percent of AD develops in people older than 65. This form of AD is called "late-onset" AD, and its development and pattern of damage in the brain is similar to that of early-onset AD. The course of this disease varies from person to person, as does the rate of decline. In most people with AD, symptoms first appear after age 65.

We do not yet completely understand the causes of late-onset AD, but they probably include genetic, environmental, and lifestyle factors. Although the risk of developing AD increases with age, AD and dementia symptoms are not a part of normal aging. There are also some forms of dementia that are not related to brain diseases such as AD, but are caused by systemic abnormalities such as metabolic syndrome, in which the combination of high blood pressure, high cholesterol, and diabetes causes confusion and memory loss.

Advances in Alzheimer's Disease

- Incidence and prevalence
- Search for etiology, genetics
- Understanding pathophysiology
- Better screening tools for early recognition
- Improved diagnosis
- Developing interventions
- Behavioral conditions and management

What research is being done?
The National Institute of Neurological Disorders and Stroke (NINDS) supports basic and translational research related to AD through grants to major medical institutions across the country. Current studies are investigating how the development of beta amyloid plaques damages neurons, and how abnormalities in tau proteins create the characteristic neurofibrillary tangles of AD. Other research is exploring the impact of risk factors associated with the development of AD, such as pre-existing problems with blood flow in the blood vessels of the brain. Most importantly, the NINDS supports a number of studies that are developing and testing new and novel therapies that can relieve the symptoms of AD and potentially lead to a cure.

Alzheimer's Disease Prevalence
 Alzheimer's disease is the most prevalent cause of dementia, accounting for between 55% 65% of all cases of dementia. While there were fewer than 3 million cases of Alzheimer's disease diagnosed in the United States in 1980, the Census Bureau predicts there will be more than 10 million American citizens with Alzheimer's disease by the year 2050. The prevalence of this disease is believed to double with every five year period of time between the ages of 65 and 85 years old.

Some researchers separate Alzheimer's disease into senile and pre-senile forms, although the two disorders actually represent the same pathological process. However, the early-onset type (onset before the age of 65) of Alzheimer's disease is usually associated with a more rapid course of progression than the later-onset type.

Alzheimer's disease affects women at a rate of 3 to 1 over men (although the reasons are unknown). Also, at least one study has suggested dementia, including Alzheimer's disease, is more common in black then white American women. Interestingly enough, comparison of population studies in various countries show distinctly similar prevalence rates.

Alzheimer's Disease Cause
The cause and pathogenesis of Alzheimer's disease is unknown. It is believed that multiple causative pathways are likely involved in this disorder. There have been many hypothesis regarding the cause and progression of Alzheimer's disease including genetic factors, slow or unconventional viruses, defective membrane metabolism, endogenous toxins, autoimmune disorders, and neurotoxicity of such trace elements as aluminum and mercury.

It is known that the brains of individuals with Alzheimer's disease contain senile plaques, neurofibrillary tangles, and Hirano's bodies. There is a deterioration of nerve cells, but the atrophy seen on neural diagnostic examination may be more the result shrinkage of neurons and the loss of dendritic spines then of the actual neuronal loss. Certain parts of the brain, such as the association cortex demonstrate the most apparent changes, with early decay in the primary motor and sensory areas being relatively spared from these changes. Cholinergic abnormalities are exhibited in the neurochemicals of the brain. There is a significant decrease in acetylcholine in most individuals along with decreased immunological activity of somatostatin and corticotropin-releasing factors. The enzyme required for acetylcholine synthesis, choline acetyltransferase, is also significantly reduced. Other studies seem to suggest involvement of the noradrenergic and serotonergic systems in later-onset Alzheimer's disease and reduced gamma-aminobutyric acid (GABA). Although it is a well-known fact that the involvement of cholinergic transmission along the hippocampus and nucleus basalis essential to the ability to learn new information, it is believed that many of the symptoms of Alzheimer's disease are not totally explained on the basis of cholinergic abnormalities. Investigators continue to examine a variety of other potential causative or contributing factors.

Researchers have also investigated the role of beta-amyloid protein in Alzheimer's disease, and some even believe that this material, a significant component of all plaques, is a major contributor to the neurodegenerative changes associated with the disease, possibly both initiating and promoting the disease process. This assertion is also supported by genetic studies of families with heritable forms of presenile dementia, which seem to indicate that disease occurrence is linked to mutations involving beta-amyloid-related systems. Also, some investigators have focused on the neurofibrillary tangles and the identification of a major component of its helical filament, the tau protein. These researchers have considered the possibility that modification of tau protein, predominantly by phosphorylation, is an important feature in the development of Alzheimer's disease.

Prevalence of AD

- Estimated 4 million cases in US (2000)
  - (2000 - 46 million individuals over 60 y/o)
- Estimated 500,000 new cases per year
- Increase with age   (prevalence)
  - 1% of 60 - 65 (10.7m) = 107,000
  - 2% of 65 - 70 (9.4m) = 188,000
  - 4% of 70 - 75 (8.7m) = 350,000
  - 8% of 75 - 80 (7.4m) = 595,000
  - 16% of 80 - 85 (5.0m) = 800,000

Alzheimer's Disease Prevalence Rates Rise

The Alzheimer's Association today reports that in 2007 there are now more than 5 million people in the United States living with Alzheimer's disease. This number includes 4.9 million people over the age of 65 and between 200,000 and 500,000 people under age 65 with early onset Alzheimer's disease and other dementias. This is a 10 percent increase from the previous prevalence nationwide estimate of 4.5 million.

The greatest risk factor for Alzheimer's is increasing age, and with 78 million baby boomers beginning to turn 60 last year, it is estimated that someone in America develops Alzheimer's every 72 seconds; by mid-century someone will develop Alzheimer's every 33 seconds.

These new estimates, as well as other data concerning the disease and its effects, are issued today as hundreds of advocates from across the country gather in the nation's capitol for the Alzheimer's Association's annual Public Policy Forum. The report titled, 2007 Alzheimer's disease Facts and Figures, is being released at a hearing today chaired by Senator Barbara Mikulski. Senators Barbara Mikulski and Christopher Bond and Representatives Edward Markey and Christopher Smith have introduced bipartisan legislation to address problems identified in the Association's report. The Association's report details the escalation of Alzheimer's disease which now is the seventh leading cause of death in the country and the fifth leading cause of death for those over age 65. It also offers numerous statistics that convey the burden that Alzheimer's imposes on individuals, families, state and federal governments, businesses, and the nation's health care system. For example:

- Without a cure or effective treatments to delay the onset or progression of the Alzheimer's, the prevalence could soar to 7.7 million people with the disease by 2030, which is more than the population of 140 of the 236 United Nations countries.

- By mid-century, the number of people with Alzheimer's is expected to grow to as many as 16 million, more than the current total population of New York City, Los Angeles, Chicago and Houston combined.
- As the prevalence impact of Alzheimer's grows, so does the cost to the nation. The direct and indirect costs of Alzheimer's and other dementias amount to more than $148 billion annually, which is more than the annual sales of any retailer in the world excluding Wal-Mart.

"Alzheimer's disease Facts and Figures clearly shows the tremendous impact this disease is having on the nation; and with the projected growth of the disease, the collective impact on individuals, families, Medicare, Medicaid, and businesses will be even greater," says Harry Johns, President, and CEO of the Alzheimer's Association. "However there is hope. There are currently nine drugs in Phase III clinical trials for Alzheimer's several of which show great promise to slow or stop the progression of the disease. This, combined with advancements in diagnostic tools, has the potential to change the landscape of Alzheimer's."

According to the latest statistics from the Centers for Disease Control and Prevention, from 2000-2004 death rates have declined for most major diseases -- heart disease (-8 percent), breast cancer (-2.6 percent), prostate cancer (-6.3 percent) and stroke (-10.4 percent), while Alzheimer's disease deaths continue to trend upward, increasing 33 percent during that period.

"We must make the fight against Alzheimer's a national priority before it's too late. The absence of effective disease modifying drugs, coupled with an aging population, makes Alzheimer's the health care crisis of the 21st century," Johns said.

Medicare currently spends nearly three times as much for people with Alzheimer's and other dementias than for the average Medicare beneficiary. Medicare costs are projected to double from $91 billion in 2005 to more than $189 billion by 2015, more than the current gross national product of 86 percent of the world's countries. In 2005, state and federal Medicaid spending for nursing home and home care for people with Alzheimer's and other dementias was estimated at $21 billion; that number is projected to increase to $27 billion by 2015.

The new report also highlights the impact that Alzheimer's has on states with more than 6 in 10 (62%) having double digit growth in prevalence by the end of the decade. In addition, Alaska (+47%), Colorado (+47%), Utah (+45%), Wyoming (+43%), Nevada (+38%), Idaho (+37%), Oregon (+33%), and Washington (+33%) will experience increases ranging from one-third to one-half. The states with the largest numbers of deaths due to Alzheimer's disease in 2003 were (1) California, (2) Florida, (3) Texas, (4) Pennsylvania, and (5) Ohio.

The Alzheimer's Association is the first and largest voluntary health organization dedicated to finding prevention methods, treatments and an eventual cure for Alzheimer's. For more than 25 years, the Association has provided reliable information and care consultation; created services for families; increased funding for dementia research; and influenced public policy changes.

Alzheimer's Prevalence Tops Five Million in U.S.
Source: (University of Pennsylvannia School of Medicine, 2007)

In its *2007 Alzheimer's Facts and Figures*, the association estimated that 2.4 million people age from the ages of 75 to 84 years -- 19% of the all U.S. adults in this age range -- have Alzheimer's. Among Americans ages 85 and older, an estimated 42%, or 2.2 million people, are living with dementia, the report stated. Alzheimer's Association estimated that there are 300,000 Americans ages 65 to 74 with Alzheimer's (2% of the U.S. population for this age range). There are approximately 500,000 Americans younger than 65 with Alzheimer's or another dementia. It is estimated that at least 200,000 of these people younger than 65 have early-onset Alzheimer's The other early-onset dementia cases may be attributable to Lewy body disease, frontotemporal disease, normal pressure hydrocephalus, Parkinson's disease, or Creutzfeldt-Jakob, the report said. The prevalence estimates were derived primarily from a single Chicago research team's studies in 2003 that were extrapolated to 2007, at the request of the Alzheimer's Association. "The dramatic rise in Alzheimer's underscores that this disease has the ability to undermine the entire U.S. healthcare system," asserted Stephen McConnell, Ph.D., the vice president of advocacy and public policy for the Alzheimer's Association, in a statement. "Looking just at Medicare and Medicaid, if we could find an intervention that could delay onset or slow progression of the disease, in short order spending on Alzheimer's could decline by more than $60 billion, with even larger savings every year thereafter." Other findings in the study included:

Deaths attributable to Alzheimer's disease increased 32.8% from 2000 to 2004. In contrast, deaths from heart disease, breast and prostate cancers and stroke all declined over the same period.

Direct and indirect costs of Alzheimer's and other dementias amount to more than $148 billion annually.

Medicare spent $91 billion on beneficiaries with Alzheimer's and other dementias in 2005, a figure that is projected to more than double to $189 billion by 2015.

The report also contained a special section on the burdens of caregiving, noting that nearly 10 million Americans care for a person with Alzheimer's or other dementia, and about one-third of the caregivers are 60 or older. Unpaid caregivers provided an estimated 8.5 billion hours of care, valued at nearly $83 billion in 2005. "A million of these caregivers in California, for example, provided an estimated $8.5 billion of care that year," the report noted. "Even Rhode Island, the smallest state, had almost 37,000 caregivers of people with Alzheimer's and other dementias, and those caregivers provided 32 million hours of care worth $310.7 million." In a state-by-state breakdown of prevalence projected out to 2010, only New York and the District of Columbia are expected to see declines in residents living with Alzheimer's disease compared with the year 2000.

The incidence figures were converted to prevalence estimates, adjusted for education and other factors, and applied to U.S. Census Bureau population figures for the year 2000 and U.S. Census Bureau projections for the years 2010, 2020, 2030, 2040 and 2050 (Hebert et. al., 2003)." " The researchers calculated the prevalence of Alzheimer's disease in each state by combining the incidence figures from the Chicago study with U. S. Census Bureau figures for the population of the state in 2000, U.S. Census Bureau projections for the state for 2010, and state-specific adjustments for gender, race, education, and mortality (Hebert et. al., 2004)." He association said that in early 2007 at its request the researchers calculated the national prevalence of Alzheimer's disease in people age 65 and over for that year, using linear extrapolation from their previous published estimates for 2000 and 2010. Additional incidence figures came from a published study of the incidence of Alzheimer's disease in stratified random samples of residents age 65 and over in east Boston (Hebert et. al., 2001). Prevalence figures for people under age 65 come from a 2006 Alzheimer's Association report (Alzheimer's Association, 2006) and are based on an analysis of available data from the Health and Retirement Study and other published articles discussed in detail in the report."

Economic Impact of AD

- Two million AD patients in nursing homes
- Nursing homes cost - $120 to $160 per day
- Annualized cost of nursing homes ranges from $40,000 to $70,000 per year
- Care of AD patients costs $80 billion per year
- With lost wages of patients and families plus costs for non-nursing home patients:
  - Total costs: $120 billion annually (*American Journal of Public Health*)

Source: (Alzheimer's Facts for Health)

The overall costs of Alzheimer's disease (AD) are staggering, but not immediately meaningful to individuals and families facing the disease. In 1991, the direct costs for providing care (such as medications, doctors' fees, and nursing home care) for Alzheimer's disease patients in the United States were approximately 20.6 billion dollars. Indirect costs, such as loss of productivity of those suffering Alzheimer's disease and loss of productivity of those caring for these individuals, added an additional 55.7 billion dollars, to yield a grand total cost of 76.3 billion (1991) dollars. The current estimate is over 100 billion dollars a year.

More to the point for individual families, the largest part of the direct costs of caring for Alzheimer's disease patients comes from nursing home care. The average cost of nursing home care has been estimated by the Alzheimer's Association to be $42,000 per year with cost exceeding $70,000 per year in some areas of the country. The Association also estimated the average lifetime cost per patient to be $174,000. For comparison, the average cost for college undergraduate education is $22,520 per year (*Digest of Education Statistics*, 2002).

Whether considering global, family or individual numbers, the cost of Alzheimer's disease is enormous. Often these costs far exceed the resources of individuals with AD and their families.

The Economic Burden of Alzheimer's Disease Care
Source: (D. Rice, 1992)

This study examines total formal and informal care costs attributable to Alzheimer's disease for persons living in the community and in institutions. The total cost of caring for an Alzheimer's client in northern California is approximately $47,000 per year whether the client lives at home or in a nursing home, but the cost breakdown differs in the two settings. For community-resident patients, three-fourths of the total cost represents an imputed value for unpaid informal care compared with 12 percent for institutionalized patients. Formal services are financed primarily by individuals and their families. Over 60 percent of the services provided to patients in either care setting were paid out of pocket. With projected increases in the number of persons at risk of developing Alzheimer's disease, the economic impact of the disease on future long-term care costs will be significant.

Etiology

- Age (initial genesis vs response to stress)
  - Bigger factor than for mortality
  - Design in a plastic (memory) system, energy demands
  - Stressor response (adequate repair mechanisms)
    - Trauma (head injury), vascular (stroke), surgery, loss, grief, etc.
- Genetics (amyloid related)
  - Familial, early onset: APP (21), PS (14, 1) (less than 5%)
  - Late onset: APOE e4 (ch19) (?50% of AD)
    - relation to brain cholesterol metabolism?
    - APOE e2 may be most protective
  - Many other candidate genes

Source: (Itzhak, 1994)
Inherited cases of Alzheimer's disease (AD) comprise only a very small proportion of the total. The remainder is of unknown etiopathogenesis, but they are very probably multifactorial in origin. This article describes studies on four possible factors: aluminum; viruses--in particular, herpes simplex type I virus (HSV1); defective DNA repair; and head trauma. Specific problems associated with aluminum, such as inadvertent contamination and its insolubility, have led to some controversy over its usage. Nonetheless, the effects of aluminum on animals and neuronal cells in culture have been studied intensively. Changes in protein structure and location in the cell are described, including the finding in this laboratory of a change in tau resembling that in AD neurofibrillary tangles, and also the lack of appreciable binding of aluminum to DNA. As for HSV1, there has previously been uncertainty about whether HSV1 DNA is present in human brain. Work in this laboratory using polymerase chain reaction has shown that HSV1 DNA is present in many normal aged brains and AD brains, but is absent in brains from younger people. Studies on DNA damage and repair in AD and normal cells are described, and finally, the possible involvement of head trauma is discussed.

The five main etiological theories of AD are reviewed:
- Genetic.
- Toxic.
- Infectious Agent.
- Immune Function.
- Trauma.

Genetic

In five studies of first degree relatives of AD cases, four have shown an increased AD frequency. In a study with age of onset of AD over 70; statistical correlation could not be found. This has created a belief that there might be two types of AD, familial and random. (Chandra et.al., 1987) Heston et.al., 1981 also found risk similar to the general population for probands over 70. Chandra further states that an aggregation of cases within families does not delineate inherited factors; that the shared environment of families could be the explanation.

Toxic
Several studies have shown that rabbits and cats (Crapper et.al., 1973) exposed to toxic levels of Aluminum (Al) develop NT. These NT are a little bit different from those found in AD patients. Data on elevated Al in AD patients has been conflicting and many cases show cerebrospinal fluid and serum Al levels to be normal in AD patients. Dialysis Dementia, a disease of elevated Al has no NT.

Infectious Agent
It has been conclusively shown that other degenerative neurological illnesses, such as Kuru, Creutzfeld~acob Disease (CJD), Gerstmann-Straussler syndrome, and Scrapie in animals are transmissible dementias caused by Prions, (Harrow et.al., 1986) curious subviral agents with no nucleic acid (Prusiner, 1984A). These syndromes contain some degree of amyloid plaques like AD but not the NT.

Immune Function
Immune function abnormalities are common in AD patients. Serum protein variances, impaired cellular immune responses, and elevated levels of brain antibodies are some of these. (Jenike, 1985) The altered immune function could explain the presence of amyloid in senile plaques. And as mentioned earlier there is also a Somatin-like immunoreactivity involved in the plaques of AD. There is still insufficient evidence to draw any definite conclusion about immune related causes of AD (Jenike, 1985) the immune function theory is still the least researched; in view of the incompleteness the other etiologies provide perhaps the answer will turn up in the immune function area. Progress is being made; an immunoreactive undecapeptide called Substance P has also been found in senile plaques (Beal, 1987) which make the immune function theory more attractive.

Trauma
People with head trauma or subdural hematoma, and thyroid disease are more prone to develop AD (Shalat et.al., 1987; Graves et.al., 1990; Gedye et.al., 1989). Also Parkinson's disease, brain tumors, Multiple Sclerosis, Epilepsy, and mental retardation correlate with AD (Chandra et.al., 1987) Depression and the presence of extrapyramidal signs of psychosis also lead to greater AD disability (Stern et.al., 1987). This could mean that the geriatric condition in general creates a susceptibility to AD from an as yet unknown cause.

Discussion
Significant evidence supports each model of AD discussed, with none being mutually exclusive of the other (Bradley, 1990); making AD appear as a complex multi-factor syndrome. Recently all the same topical factors were considered as the pathogenesis of cancer; and all researchers were deemed correct. The time has approached to isolate and go beyond Amoroso - Alzheimer's Noetic Journal V. 2 No. 2, April, 1999 237 the "elephantness" of AD. (Wurtman, 1985) This metaphor is of five blind men confronted by an elephant: One thinks of the tail as a rope; another leg as a tree; the trunk as a hose, the body as a wall, and the fifth thinks the ear is a large fan.

The Current lens through which unification of the elephant is being attempted is that of premature aging. (Bosman & Bartholomeus, 1991; Rabinowe et.al., 1989; Bertoni-Freddari, 1988; Masters & Beyreuther, 1988).

The nature of aging is an extremely difficult concept for science; however, aging has been postulated as being either genetically driven or of a stochastic process. It is not known if either or both is correct (Gershon, 1988).

Only weak correlational evidence supports programmed senescence. Cell cultures die off after about 50 doublings for human cells; proportionally less doublings for shorter lifespan animals, for example embryonic fibroblasts from rats and chickens double only about 15 times. Interestingly cells from midlife humans double only about 25 times (Hayflick, 1968).

The most significant of the random negative factors considered is free radical damage. The Harman "Free Radical Theory of Aging" is over 30 years old. (Gershon, 1988) There is free radical etiology support for each "elephant" factor.

(Forster & Harbans, 1991; Cutler, 1991; Evans et.al., 1991; Volicer & Crino, 1990; Bergtold, 1988) A correlation has been found between endogenous antioxidants and the lifespan of mammals; suggesting that oxidative stress is less in mammals with longer lifespans. (Cutler, 1991) This issue is being tested by measuring 8~hydroxydeoxyguanosine per deoxyguanosine levels in liver DNA and urine (Bergtold, 1988). The author suggests that if free radicals do play an additional putative role in the pathogenesis of AD; this urine biomarker could be also studied comparing AD patients with normal human population.

Etiology

- Relation to vascular factors, cholesterol, BP

- Education (design vs protection)

- Environment - diet, exercise, smoking

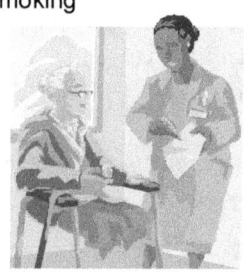

Education 'Reduces Alzheimer's Effects'
Source: (News, 2003)

People who spend years studying at university may be inadvertently protecting themselves against severe Alzheimer's disease, a study suggests:

- Scientists in the United States have found evidence to suggest that a formal education protects against the more devastating aspects of the disease.

- They have discovered a direct link between the amount of time spent studying and the loss of memory and learning skills in people with Alzheimer's.

- The scientists believe that a long history of education may enable the brain to cope better with the effects of the disease.

Cognitive Tests
Dr. David Bennett and colleagues at Rush Presbyterian-St Luke's Medical Center in Chicago examined the brains of 130 people who had been diagnosed with Alzheimer's before they died. Their education levels varied although 90% had gone to college. This ranged from a few years of undergraduate study to high levels of postgraduate work.

Education May Make the Brain More Adaptable and Flexible
All of these people had undergone tests about eight months before their death. The tests examined their cognitive abilities - their ability to memorize and process information and their ability to accurately reach for objects within their visual field. They found that the longer people spent in formal education the better they performed in these tests. This was irrespective of the amount of amyloid plaques - proteins which clump together to kill cells - in their brains. These plaques are known to cause Alzheimer's.

Writing in the journal Neurology, the scientists suggested that years of education could help to build up a reserve which can help the brain to cope better in the event of Alzheimer's disease. "[Education] may make the brain more adaptable and flexible," Dr.

Bennett said. Dr. Neil Buckholtz, head of the US National Institute on Aging, backed that view.

"These findings give us additional insight into the long-known but well understood link between education and everyday memory and learning ability," he said. "It may be that education permits the brain already affected by the pathology of Alzheimer's disease to work around that damage and allow an individual to function at a higher level."

Story from BBC NEWS:
http://news.bbc.co.uk/go/pr/fr/-/1/hi/health/3014582.stm
Published: 2003/06/23 20:49:22 GMT

Relative Risk Factors for Alzheimer's Disease

- Family history of dementia
- Family history - Downs
- Family history - Parkinson's
- Maternal age > 40 years
- Head trauma (with loss of conscious)
- History of depression
- History of hypothyroidism
- History of severe headache

Roca, 1994, t'Veldt, 2002

Source: (Alz.org)

Age

The greatest known risk factor for Alzheimer's is increasing age. Most individuals with the disease are 65 or older. The likelihood of developing Alzheimer's doubles about every five years after age 65. After age 85, the risk reaches nearly 50 percent.

Family History
Another risk factor is family history. Research has shown that those who have a parent, brother or sister, or child with Alzheimer's are more likely to develop Alzheimer's. The risk increases if more than one family member has the illness. When diseases tend to run in families, either heredity (genetics) or environmental factors or both may play a role.

Genetics (Heredity)
Scientists know genes are involved in Alzheimer's. There are two categories of genes that can play a role in determining whether a person develops a disease. Alzheimer genes have been found in both categories:

1) Risk genes increase the likelihood of developing a disease, but do not guarantee it will happen. Scientists have so far identified one Alzheimer risk gene called apolipoprotein E-e4 (APOE-e4). APOE-e4 is one of three common forms of the APOE gene; the others are APOE-e2 and APOE-e3. APOE provides the blueprint for one of the proteins that carries cholesterol in the bloodstream.

Everyone inherits a copy of some form of APOE from each parent. Those who inherit one copy of APOE-e4 have an increased risk of developing Alzheimer's. Those who inherit two copies have an even higher risk, but not a certainty. Scientists do not yet know how APOE-e4 raises risk. In addition to raising risk, APOE-e4 may tend to make symptoms appear at a younger age than usual.

2) Deterministic genes directly cause a disease, guaranteeing that anyone who inherits them will develop the disorder.
Scientists have found rare genes that directly cause Alzheimer's in only a few hundred extended families worldwide.

When Alzheimer's disease is caused by deterministic genes, it is called "familial Alzheimer's disease," and many family members in multiple generations are affected. True familial Alzheimer's accounts for less than 5 percent of cases.

Genetic tests are available for both APOE-e4 and the rare genes that directly cause Alzheimer's. However, health professionals do not currently recommend routine genetic testing for Alzheimer's disease. Testing for APOE-e4 is sometimes included as a part of research studies.

Risk Factors able to be Influenced

Age, family history, and heredity are all risk factors we cannot change. Now, research is beginning to reveal clues about other risk factors we may be able to influence.

Head Injury: There appears to be a strong link between serious head injury and future risk of Alzheimer's. Protect your head by buckling your seat belt, wearing your helmet when participating in sports, and "fall-proofing" your home.

Heart-Head Connection: Some of the strongest evidence links brain health to heart health. Your brain is nourished by one of your body's richest networks of blood vessels. Every heartbeat pumps about 20 to 25 percent of your blood to your head, where brain cells use at least 20 percent of the food and oxygen your blood carries.

The risk of developing Alzheimer's or vascular dementia appears to be increased by many conditions that damage the heart or blood vessels. These include high blood pressure, heart disease, stroke, diabetes, and high cholesterol. Work with your doctor to monitor your heart health and treat any problems that arise.

General Healthy Aging: Other lines of evidence suggest that strategies for overall healthy aging may help keep the brain healthy and may even offer some protection against developing Alzheimer has or related diseases. Try to keep your weight within recommended guidelines, avoid tobacco and excess alcohol, stay socially connected, and exercise both your body and mind.

```
┌─────────────────────────────────────────────────────┐
│                                                       │
│     Diagnostic Criteria For Dementia Of The           │
│     Alzheimer Type     (DSM-IV, APA, 1994)            │
│                                                       │
│   A.  Multiple Cognitive Deficits                     │
│        1. Memory Impairment                           │
│        2. Other Cognitive Impairment                  │
│   B.  Deficits Impair Social/Occupational             │
│   C.  Course Shows Gradual Onset And Decline          │
│   D.  Deficits Are Not Due to:                        │
│        1. Other CNS Conditions                        │
│        2. Substance Induced Conditions                │
│   E.  Do Not Occur Exclusively during Delirium        │
│   F.  Not Due to Another Psychiatric Disorder         │
│                                                       │
└─────────────────────────────────────────────────────┘
```

Source: (About.com, 2008)
Alzheimer's disease is difficult to diagnose, and it is best when a team of professionals -- including a neurologist, neuropsychologist, geriatrician, and possibly others -- works together to arrive at an accurate diagnosis. A total diagnostic workup includes a medical history, imaging procedures, and neuropsychological testing, as well as other procedures depending on the individual's presentation.

- *Aphasia* -- a deterioration of language abilities, which can manifest in several ways
- *Apraxia* -- difficulty executing motor activities, even though movement, senses, and the ability to understand what is being asked are still intact
- *Agnosia* -- an impaired ability to recognize or identify objects, even though sensory abilities are intact

Problems with *executive functioning*, such as planning tasks, organizing projects, or carrying out goals in the proper sequence

In order to meet the criteria for Alzheimer's disease, the deficits must affect one's ability to hold a job or volunteer position, fulfill domestic responsibilities, and/or maintain social relationships. The deficits must also represent a significant decline from the person's previous level of functioning.

Alzheimer's disease involves a gradual onset and progressive worsening of symptoms. In order to receive a diagnosis of Alzheimer's, the deficits cannot be due to another medical condition, such as Parkinson's disease, thyroid problems, or alcoholism. Similarly, the symptoms cannot occur exclusively during an episode of delirium, or be better explained by a psychological disorder such as depression or schizophrenia.

New Diagnostic Criteria for Alzheimer's Disease
An international group of Alzheimer's disease (AD) experts have proposed new criteria for the research diagnosis of the condition, as they argue the existing criteria are out of date due to unprecedented growth of scientific knowledge in the field. The proposal is put forward in a Position Paper published early online and in the August edition of The Lancet Neurology.

AD is a neurodegenerative disease characterized by progressive cognitive deterioration, together with declining activities of daily living and by neuropsychiatric symptoms or behavioral changes. It is the most common form of dementia.

The existing criteria were published in 1984 by the National Institute of Neurological Disorders and Stroke-Alzheimer Disease and Related Disorders (NINCDS-ADRDA) working group. Dr. Bruno Dubois, Salpêtrière Hospital, Paris, France, and colleagues, say: "[These existing criteria] are the prevailing diagnostic standards in research; however they have now fallen behind the unprecedented growth of scientific knowledge. Distinctive and reliable biomarkers of AD are now available through structural MRI, molecular neuroimaging with PET*, and cerebrospinal fluid analyses."

To meet the new criteria for probable AD, patients must show progressive memory loss over more than six months, plus at least one or more of the supportive biomarker criteria. These include: atrophy in a particular part of the brain shown by MRI, abnormal biomarker proteins in the cerebrospinal fluid, a specific pattern on PET of the brain, and a genetic mutation for AD within the immediate family. The authors say: "These new criteria are centered on a clinical core of early and significant episodic memory impairment...the timeliness of these criteria is highlighted by the many drugs in development that are directed at changing pathogenesis."

The researchers add that validation studies are required to advance the new criteria and optimize their sensitivity, specificity, and accuracy. They conclude: "When effective disease-modifying medications are available, the argument for such biologically based studies will be even more compelling. "These proposed criteria move away from the traditional two-step approach of first identifying dementia according to degree of functional disability, and then specifying its cause. Rather, they aim to define the clinical, biochemical, structural, and metabolic presence of AD."

In an accompanying comment, Dr. Norman Foster, Center for Alzheimer's Care, Department of Neurology, and University of Utah, USA says: "We should seize this opportunity to reopen the discussion of Alzheimer's disease diagnosis. The time is right to use the advanced technology at our disposal to improve the early, accurate diagnosis of dementia and develop more effective treatments."

Neuropathology in Alzheimer's Disease: Awaking from a Hundred-Year-Old Dream
Source: (Science AAAS, 2006)

Introduction

One hundred years ago, the German psychiatrist and neuropathologist Alois Alzheimer gave a lecture that made him famous, in which he identified a disease of the cerebral cortex, namely, Alzheimer's disease (AD). In individuals with this condition, the cerebral cortex was thinner than normal, and senile plaques, previously only encountered in elderly people, were found in the brain along with neurofibrillary tangles (NFTs) (1) (see Honig and Chin Case Study). Amyloid- (A) and the microtubule-associated protein tau, major constituents of extracellular senile plaques and intraneuronal NFTs, respectively, are among the best studied proteins in all of neurobiology and figure centrally into much of the research dedicated to AD (see "Detangling Alzheimer's Disease"). Although this emphasis is not surprising, as the pathological diagnosis of AD is dependent on the quantity of A and tau deposits within cortical gray matter (2, 3), we suggest that this strict linkage of diagnostic and mechanistic views is misleading, particularly in the case of neurodegenerative disease.

Neuropathological changes in subjects with dementia are, by definition, end-stage phenomena. Although such changes allow case characterization and lend themselves to disease classification and modeling, the lesions themselves are not etiological. They are pathognomonic but not pathogenic. This truth would appear to be self-evident, yet the medical and scientific literature suggests otherwise. It is now customary to view plaques in AD as primary etiological, neurotoxic lesions, such that by removing them through immunotherapy, clinical improvement may result. The foundation for this line of thinking lies in the existence of rare kindreds (in which individuals are at high risk for developing AD) with mutations in A , or mutations believed to affect the processing of A , and then the extrapolation of concepts relevant to the inherited condition to sporadic disease. We believe that this overall construct ignores early events that are more critical to the onset and progression of sporadic disease. In this Perspective, we present an alternative hypothesis for the role of A and tau deposition in AD that may herald a paradigm shift in our views of neurodegenerative diseases.

The long-held notion that pathological lesions in neurodegenerative diseases provide direct insight into etiology may be a fundamental misconception. The observed decrease in oxidative damage with A and tau accumulation suggests that senile plaques and NFTs are manifestations of cellular adaptation. Therapeutic strategy aimed solely at eliminating A or tau may therefore be directed against a biochemical process that is more physiological than pathological and therefore unlikely to produce the desired results. We further suggest that the classical notion of the pathological hallmarks as signifying neurodegenerative disease should be reorganized into a modern framework that recognizes the difference between cause and effect. Only through such an effort will the greatest potential for continued diagnostic and therapeutic advances be realized.

Biopsychosocial Systems
Affected by AD
(all related to neuroplasticity)

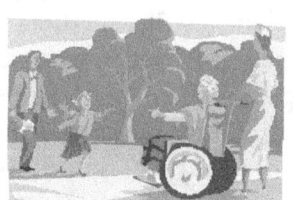

- Social Systems
  - Instrumental ADLs - Early
  - Basic ADLs - Late
- Psychological Systems
  - Primary Loss Of Memory
  - Later Loss Of Learned Skills
- Neuronal Memory Systems

Early-Alzheimer's Disease Program Focuses on Support, Enrichment
Source: (O'Brien, 2007)

In the early stages of Alzheimer's disease, people experience mild memory loss and confusion. These challenges are significant, but people often maintain much of their normal capability and spirit. Now, a specialized support group program is being formed at the UCSF Memory and Aging Center to help patients learn how to live with the disease and to help family members grieve and adjust. The program, co-sponsored by the Alzheimer's Association of Northern California and Northern Nevada, is currently enrolling participants.

"Some 2.5 million patients in the United States currently have a diagnosis of early-stage Alzheimer's disease," says Bruce Miller, MD, director of the UCSF Memory and Aging Center. "Their lives, and that of their families, could be enriched by this program."

"People diagnosed early in the course of the disease often become isolated and stigmatized, even though they may be quite healthy and functional for a number of years," says Rosalie Gearhart, RN,

MSN, a nurse in the UCSF Center. While many can no longer work, they typically live at home, care for themselves, and continue to enjoy many pleasurable activities.

"The support group helps to maintain emotional well-being, social support, and intellectual stimulation," explains Robyn Yale, LCSW, a licensed clinical social worker. Yale, a consultant to the Alzheimer's Association, developed the early stage Alzheimer's disease support group model and has helped implement it across the United States and internationally.

As a 79-year-old man from another Bay Area support group declared, Yale recalls, "I want people to know I have a lot of life left!"

In the support group, patients receive information, share feelings, and experiences with others in a similar situation, and learn coping strategies. "Issues in common include losing one's driver's license and adjusting to increasing dependency and changes in relationships with family and friends," says Yale. "Patients also discuss what they are experiencing in their lives, and how to sustain their capabilities for as long as possible."

Family members of those with early Alzheimer's disease meet in a separate support group at the same time and location. They focus on care-giving issues unique to the beginning of the illness, such as restructuring household responsibilities and determining when to assist the person with Alzheimer's disease and when to encourage independence. Occasionally, the concurrent support groups meet jointly, allowing all participants to interact.

"Patients have reported an increased understanding and acceptance of memory loss and improved mood and morale from the camaraderie of support groups," says Yale, who is helping establish the program at UCSF.

Likewise, she says, family members report feeling less isolated, gaining knowledge about coping and realizing that planning now for the future needs to include the person with the disease, which will no longer be possible in Alzheimer's disease's later stages. Additionally, caregivers learn sooner than they might otherwise, she says, about the range of services available throughout the course of the disease.

To join the group, individuals must have a diagnosis of dementia, be informed of—and at least occasionally be able to acknowledge—the illness, have good communication and social skills, and want to participate in the group.

To be screened for potential participation in the program at the UCSF Memory and Aging Center, patients or their families should contact Heather Gray at the Alzheimer's Association of Northern California and Northern Nevada at (650) 623-3133.

The Alzheimer's Association began sponsoring the support group programs in the Bay Area in 1994, says Yale. There are now programs in San Rafael, Berkeley, Lafayette, San Jose, and San Mateo. The San Francisco group is re-starting after a hiatus of several years. For enrollment in programs outside of San Francisco, contact the Alzheimer's Association of Northern California and Northern Nevada at (800) 272-3900.

UCSF is a leading university that advances health worldwide by conducting advanced biomedical research, educating graduate students in the life sciences and health professions, and providing complex client care.

Social Support is Key for Alzheimer's Caregivers
Source: (Fisher Center for Alzheimer's Research Foundation, 2006)

Maintaining a close network of family and friends who can be called on for emotional support may be key to managing day-to-day care in those who care for a loved one with Alzheimer's disease at home, researchers report. The findings are based on results from the long-running study led by Dr. Mary Mittelman at the Silberstein Institute at the New York University School of Medicine. Caregivers who tended to a husband or wife with

Alzheimer's disease felt generally less stressed and more satisfied when they were educated about the disease and provided with ongoing counseling and support services. Strong emotional support, frequent interactions, and visits from others, and a large network of friends and family who could be called on all appeared to boost satisfaction and enhance day-to-day coping skills.

Some five million Americans care for a loved one with Alzheimer's disease at home, a burden that can take a big toll on health and well-being. Many such caregivers feel isolated from family and friends, and stress levels are likely to rise as symptoms grow more severe with time and the requirements of care increase.

At the NYU Silberstein Aging and Dementia Research Center, researchers have been providing a targeted program of counseling and support in the NYU Spouse-Caregiving Intervention Study, the longest running research project of its kind. The NYU approach employs several key strategies designed to help friends and family cope with the stress of caring for someone with Alzheimer's disease. Components of the program include:

> 1) Education of caregivers and family members about Alzheimer's disease, its effects on the client, how best to manage care and respond to symptoms, and how to improve social support for caregivers.

> 2) Counseling and ongoing support for the care partner and family members, including both individual and family counseling, encouragement for caregivers to join support groups, and telephone counseling for the caregiver and other family members when needed.

> 3) Improving social support and reducing family conflict to help the caregiver withstand the hardships of caregiving and to help family members understand the primary caregiver's needs, and how best to be helpful.

Counseling can play an important role in improving general mental health in people who care for someone with Alzheimer's disease. When social support is available through support groups and professional counseling, people have a chance to express positive and negative feelings about coping with hardship. Discussing problems with counselors and fellow caregivers allows people to identify needs, express those needs to other family members, and adjust to the challenges of a progressive illness like Alzheimer's.

Counseling can be especially important for those who care for a spouse with Alzheimer's disease. Such caregivers tend to be elderly themselves and often are coping with ailments that may limit their mobility or cause suffering. Many spouse caregivers may become socially isolated because they are afraid to leave their partners at home alone or to go out with their partners. Behavioral problems related to Alzheimer's, such as night wandering, incontinence, agitation, and an inability even to recognize a loved one, can be particularly trying for care partners as the disease progresses.

Wide Range of Benefits
The ongoing NYU Trial, which started in 1987, has shown that a comprehensive program of counseling and support provides a wide range of benefits for those who care for a spouse with Alzheimer's disease. Such care can delay the need for a loved one with Alzheimer's disease to enter a nursing home. It can also reduce depression in caregivers, an effect that may persist for years. Spouse caregivers were also better able to cope with behavior problems related to Alzheimer's. They also felt less isolated and more connected to their social support networks, an effect that can boost overall psychological well-being.

The current study looked at 200 spouse caregivers who were caring for a loved one with Alzheimer's disease. All were given intensive counseling and support through the NYU program. During the next five years, researchers evaluated several aspects of social support, including:

- Instrumental support, including help with day-to-day activities such as cleaning the house, moving, or bathing someone with Alzheimer's, or help with driving.
- Emotional support. This includes offering a helpful ear to confide in or a shoulder to lean on during times of need.
- Information support, including advice from doctors, counselors, and other health professionals, as well as advice from peers who have gone through similar circumstances.

The researchers found that spouse-caregivers who received comprehensive counseling and support experienced consistently higher levels of satisfaction compared to a control group that received standard support and care. The benefits began within four months of the targeted program, and continued during the five years of the study.

The spouse-caregivers who received ongoing counseling and comprehensive support felt more supported by family and friends. They also tended to call on loved ones for support, and to visit or bring them into their homes, more often. This increased social support, the researchers believe, enhanced feelings of well-being among the caregivers.

The findings underline the importance of comprehensive counseling and support, as well as of nurturing a network of family and friends who can be called on for emotional support when caring for a loved one with Alzheimer's disease. Close social ties help caregivers to feel less isolated and more connected with the world around them. Visits from close family and friends help break the isolation of caring for someone with Alzheimer's disease. Such support also gives caregivers the chance to share news, report problems, and discuss feelings.

A program of counseling and support "led to sustained higher levels of social support over a five-year period, even while the behaviors of the spouse with Alzheimer's disease changed," the researchers write. "Given the growing number of people expected to be caring for a relative with Alzheimer's disease, the evidence that the intervention also enables caregivers to become less isolated and reach out more effectively to family and friends add to its appeal as a treatment that should be widely available."

Enlisting ongoing help and support throughout the care-giving process can be critical for maintaining well-being and helping to manage the extreme demands of caring for a loved one with Alzheimer's disease.

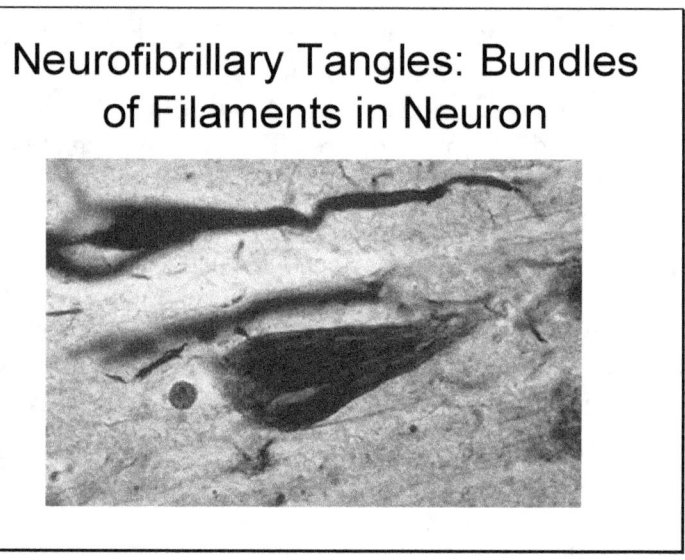

Neurofibrillary Tangles: Bundles of Filaments in Neuron

Shown is an abnormal neuron which is shown upon staining to have the neurofibrillary tangles which result in the death of the cell.

Alzheimer's disease is a degenerative disease of the brain. Understanding how the anatomy of the Alzheimer's differs from a normal brain gives us insight. It can help us cope better with the changes that happen to our loved ones as a result of this debilitating disease.

In Alzheimer's disease the appearance of the Alzheimer's affected brain is very different to a normal brain - see image.

The cerebral cortex atrophies. That means that this area of the brain shrinks and this shrinkage is dramatically different from the cerebral cortex of a normal brain. The cerebral cortex is the outer surface of the brain. It is responsible for all intellectual functioning. There are two major changes that can be observed in the brain at autopsy:

- The amount of brain substance in the folds of the brain (the gyri) is decreased
- The spaces in the folds of the brain (the sulci) are grossly enlarged.
- Microscopically there are a number of changes in the brain too.

The two major findings in the Alzheimer's brain are amyloid plaques and neurofibrillary tangles. Amyloid plaques are found outside the neurons, neurofibrillary plaques are found inside the neurons. Neurons are the nerve cells within the brain.

Plaques and tangles are found in the brains of people without Alzheimer's. It is the gross amounts of them that are significant in Alzheimer's disease.

Role of Amyloid Plaques in Alzheimer's
Amyloid plaques are mostly made up of a protein called B-amyloid protein which is itself part of a much larger protein called APP (amyloid precursor protein). These are amino acids.

We do not know what APP does. But we do know that APP is made in the cell, transported to the cell membrane, and later broken down. Two major pathways are involved in breakdown of APP (amyloid precursor protein). One pathway is normal and causes no problem. The second results in the changes seen in Alzheimer's and in some of the other dementias.

Pathway Breakdown Leading to Alzheimer's Damage
In the second breakdown pathway APP is split by enzymes B-secretes (B=beta) then y-secretes (y=gamma). Some of the fragments (called peptides) that result stick together and form a short chain called an oligomer. Oligomers are also known as

ADDL, amyloid-beta derived diffusible ligands. Oligomers of amyloid beta 42 have been shown to cause problems in the communication between neurons. Amyloid beta 42 also produces tiny fibers, or fibrils. When they stick together they form amyloid plaque. Some of these plaques can insert themselves into the membrane of the neuron cell causing substances outside the cell to leak into it, causing further damage. This damage results in a buildup of Amyloid beta 42 peptide leading to neuron dysfunction and death.

Role of Neurofibrillary Tangles in Alzheimer's
The second major finding in the Alzheimer's brain is neurofibrillary tangles. Neurofibrillary tangles are composed of a protein called tau protein. Tau proteins play a crucial role in the structure of the neuron. In people with Alzheimer's tau proteins cause abnormality through overactive enzymes resulting in the formation of neurofibrillary tangles. Neurofibrillary tangles result in the death of the cells.

Alzheimer's Brain Summary
The role of amyloid plaques and neurofibrillary tangles on the functioning of the brain is by no means fully understood. Most people with Alzheimer's disease show evidence of both plaques and tangles, but a small number of people with Alzheimer's only have plaques and some have only neurofibrillary tangles.

People with plaque only Alzheimer's show a slower rate of deterioration during their lives. People with neurofibrillary tangles are more likely to be diagnosed with frontotemporal dementia.

Research into Alzheimer's disease is finding out more and more about the anatomy and physiology of the brain. As we understand more about the role of plaques and tangles observed in the Alzheimer's brain the closer we get to a significant breakthrough and a cure for Alzheimer's disease.

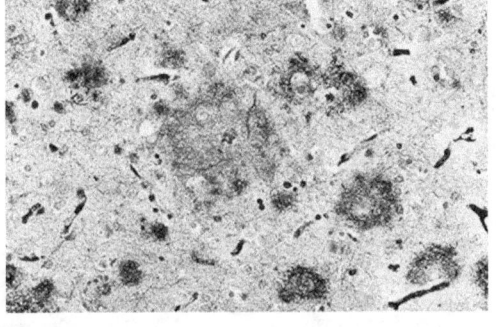

Senile Plaques: Neuritic Processes around an Amyloid Core

Shown is the other hallmark of Alzheimer's pathology: senile plaques in the cortex.

Senile plaques (syn. Neurotic plaques, senile druse, braindruse) are extracellular deposits of amyloid in the gray matter of the brain. The deposits are associated with degenerative neural structures and an abundance of microglia and astrocytes. Large numbers of senile plaques and neurofibrillary tangles are characteristic features of Alzheimer's disease.

The plaques are variable in shape and size, but are on the average 50 μm in size. (Franke, M.) In Alzheimer's disease they are primarily composed of amyloid beta peptides. These polypeptides tend to aggregate and are believed to be neurotoxic.

Verification
Senile plaques are visible in light microscopy after staining by silver, Congo red, Thioflavin, Kresylviolett, PAS-reaction, and by fluorescence and immunofluorescence microscopy.

Occurrence
Senile plaques can be found in human and animal brains (e.g. mammals and birds). From an age of 60 years (10%) to an age of

80 years (60%) the proportion of people with plaques increases approximately linearly. A small number of plaques can be due to the physiological process of aging. Women are slightly more likely to have plaques than males (Franke, M.). The plaques occur commonly in the amygdoid nucleus and the sulci of the cortex of brain.

History

Blocq and Marinesco first described plaques in the grey matter in 1892. Because of their similarity to the antinomies druses they were called druse necrosis by O. Fischer in the beginning of the 20th century. The connection of plaques and demential illness was discovered by Alzheimer in 1906. Bielschowsky supposed in 1911 the amyloid-nature of the plaques. Wisniewski denominated them neurotic plaques in 1973. The second half of the 20th century saw proposed theories of immunological and genetic factors in plaque formation (Katenkamp, Op den Velde und Stam). Statistically investigations were performed by J.A.N. Corsellis and M. Franke in the 1970s. M. Franke showed that a demential disease is likely when the number of senile plaques in the frontal cortex is more than 200/mm3. In 1985 succeeded the biochemical identification of amyloid beta. But there are more unsolved questions of formation and importance of the plaque formation.

Importance

The senile plaques are an important criterion of the neuropathological-histological verification of the Alzheimer's disease; other factors in verification include pathological neurofibrillary, tangles, atrophic brain with hydrocephalus, and other degenerative signs. The formation and the distribution of the pathological neurofibrillary have regularity (H. Braak and E. Braak) and allows to stage the disease. In combination with the occurrence of a great number of plaques the Alzheimer's disease can be diagnosed with high probability.

Genetics of AD

- In minority of cases an autosomal dominant inheritance linked to chromosome 1, 14, or 21. Associated with early onset (<60 years of age)

- Presence of an allele E4 increases risk, especially if homozygous

- AD is probably a common manifestation of multiple underlying disorders

There has been much interest about finding a genetic marker for Alzheimer's. First, let it be said that most cases of Alzheimer's disease are sporadic and not familial. In a minority of cases where it is familial, an autosomal dominant linkage has been found with chromosomes 1, 14, or 21.

There is a gene product of chromosome 19, apolipoprotein E. This is a gene product involved in the transport of cholesterol across cell membranes. APOE has been associated with an increased risk of Alzheimer 's disease. People who do not carry the allele can still get Alzheimer's disease. A consensus statement from the American College of Medical Genetics recommended against the general use of this test.

Finally, it should be said, that most researchers would probably believe that Alzheimer's disease is a common manifestation of multiple underlying disorders. It is not likely to be caused by any one metabolic abnormality.

Genetics of AD

- Presence of AD in a first degree relative is associated with a fourfold increase in risk for AD

- Lifetime risk of developing AD in first degree relatives is 50%

The Genetics of Alzheimer's Disease
Source: (National Institute on Aging)

AD is an irreversible, progressive brain disease characterized by the development of amyloid plaques and neurofibrillary tangles, the loss of connections between nerve cells in the brain, and the death of these nerve cells. AD has two types: early-onset and late-onset. Both types have genetic links.

Early-Onset AD
Early-onset AD is a rare form of AD, affecting only about 5 percent of all people who have AD. It develops in people ages 30 to 60.

Some cases of early-onset AD, called familial AD (FAD), are inherited. FAD is caused by a number of different gene mutations on chromosomes 21, 14, and 1, and each of these mutations causes abnormal proteins to be formed. Mutations on chromosome 21 cause the formation of abnormal amyloid precursor protein (APP). A mutation on chromosome 14 causes abnormal presenilin 1 to be made, and a mutation on chromosome 1 leads to abnormal presenilin 2.

Even if only one of these mutated genes is inherited from a parent, the person will almost always develop early-onset AD. This inheritance pattern is referred to as "autosomal dominant" inheritance. In other words, offspring in the same generation have a 50/50 chance of developing FAD if one of their parents had it.

Scientists know that each of these mutations causes an increased amount of the beta-amyloid protein to be formed. Beta-amyloid, a major component of AD plaques, is formed from APP.

These early-onset findings were critical because they showed that genetics were involved in AD, and they helped identify key players in the AD process. The studies also helped explain some of the variation in the age at which AD develops.

Late-Onset AD
Most cases of Alzheimer's are of the late-onset form, developing after age 60. Scientists studying the genetics of AD have found that the mutations seen in early-onset AD are not involved in this form of the disease.

Although a specific gene has not been identified as the cause of late-onset AD, one predisposing genetic risk factor does appear to increase a person's risk of developing the disease.

Scientists believe that four to seven other AD risk-factor genes exist and are using a new approach called a genome-wide association study (GWAS) to help speed the discovery process. Another possible risk-factor gene, SORL1, was discovered in 2007. This gene is involved in transporting APP within cells, and its association with AD has been identified and confirmed in three separate studies. Researchers found that when SORL1 is present at low levels or in a variant form, beta-amyloid levels increase and may harm neurons.

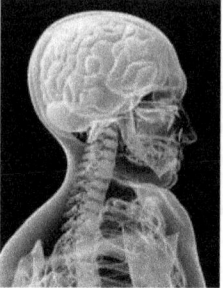

III. B. Stages of AD

Dr. Jerry Turner
IEP, Inc.

www.RCFE-CEU.com

Source: (Alzheimer's Association)
There are several different approaches to identifying the stages of Alzheimer's. The following is one such stage theory:

Stage 1:
 No impairment (normal function). Unimpaired individuals experience no memory problems and none are evident to a health care professional during a medical interview.

 Stage 2:
 Very mild cognitive decline (may be normal age-related changes or earliest signs of Alzheimer's disease).

Individuals may feel as if they have memory lapses, especially in forgetting familiar words or names or the location of keys, eyeglasses or other everyday objects. But these problems are not evident during a medical examination or apparent to friends, family, or co-workers.

Stage 3:
Mild cognitive decline. Early-stage Alzheimer's can be diagnosed in some, but not all, individuals with these symptoms

Friends, family, or co-workers begin to notice deficiencies. Problems with memory or concentration may be measurable in clinical testing or discernible during a detailed medical interview.

Common difficulties include:
- Word- or name-finding problems noticeable to family or close associates.
- Decreased ability to remember names when introduced to new people.
- Performance issues in social or work settings noticeable to family, friends or co-workers.
- Reading a passage and retaining little material.
- Losing or misplacing a valuable object.
- Decline in ability to plan or organize.

Stage 4:
Moderate cognitive decline. (Mild or early-stage Alzheimer's disease)

At this stage, a careful medical interview detects clear-cut deficiencies in the following areas:
- Decreased knowledge of recent occasions or current events.
- Impaired ability to perform challenging mental arithmetic- for example, to count backward from 75 by 7s.
- Decreased capacity to perform complex tasks, such as planning dinner for guests, paying bills and managing finances.
- Reduced memory of personal history.

The affected individual may seem subdued and withdrawn, especially in socially or mentally challenging situations.

Stage 5:
Moderately severe cognitive decline. (Moderate or mid-stage Alzheimer's disease)

Major gaps in memory and deficits in cognitive function emerge. Some assistance with day-to-day activities becomes essential. At this stage, individuals may:

- Be unable during a medical interview to recall such important details as their current address, their telephone number or the name of the college or high school from which they graduated.
- Become confused about where they are or about the date, day of the week or season.
- Have trouble with less challenging mental arithmetic; for example, counting backward from 40 by 4s or from 20 by 2s.
- Need help choosing proper clothing for the season or the occasion.
- Usually retain substantial knowledge about themselves and know their own name and the names of their spouse or children.
- Usually require no assistance with eating or using the toilet.

Stage 6:
Severe cognitive decline. (Moderately severe or mid-stage Alzheimer's disease)

Memory difficulties continue to worsen, significant personality changes may emerge, and affected individuals need extensive help with customary daily activities. At this stage, individuals may:

- Lose most awareness of recent experiences and events as well as of their surroundings.
- Recollect their personal history imperfectly, although they generally recall their own name.
- Occasionally forget the name of their spouse or primary caregiver but generally can distinguish familiar from unfamiliar faces.
- Need help getting dressed properly; without supervision, may make such errors as putting pajamas over daytime clothes or shoes on wrong feet.
- Experience disruption of their normal sleep/waking cycle.

- Need help with handling details of toileting (flushing toilet, wiping and disposing of tissue properly).
- Have increasing episodes of urinary or fecal incontinence.
- Experience significant personality changes and behavioral symptoms, including suspiciousness and delusions (for example, believing that their caregiver is an impostor); hallucinations (seeing or hearing things that are not really there); or compulsive, repetitive behaviors such as hand-wringing or tissue shredding.
- Tend to wander and become lost.

Stage 7:
Very severe cognitive decline. (Severe or late-stage Alzheimer's disease)

This is the final stage of the disease when individuals lose the ability to respond to their environment, the ability to speak and, ultimately, the ability to control movement. Frequently individuals lose their capacity for recognizable speech, although words or phrases may occasionally be uttered. Individuals need help with eating and toileting and there is general incontinence of urine. Individuals lose the ability to walk without assistance, then the ability to sit without support, the ability to smile, and the ability to hold their head up. Reflexes become abnormal and muscles grow rigid. Swallowing is impaired.

Stages of AD

- Onset and progressive course with typical loss of 3 points on MMSE each year

- Death occurring 10 - 20 years after diagnosis

How Long?
Source: (Alzheimer's Review, 2009)

The rate of progression varies widely among individuals. For some, severe dementia occurs within five years of diagnosis. For others, it can take more than a decade. On average, people with Alzheimer's live for eight to 10 years after diagnosis. Some live as long as 20 years. Most people with Alzheimer's do not die of the disease itself, but of pneumonia, a urinary tract infection, or complications from a fall.

Stage of AD - Mild

- MMSE 20-24

- Usually the first 2-3 years after diagnosis

- Primarily memory and visual-spatial deficits

- Mild difficulty with executive functions

Mild Alzheimer's Disease
Source: (Mayo Clinic)

People in the early stage of Alzheimer's may experience memory loss, lapses of judgment and subtle changes in personality. They often have decreased attention span and less motivation to complete tasks. In addition, they may resist change and new challenges, and get lost even in familiar places.

While everyone occasionally forgets words or names during conversations, this problem occurs with increasing frequency in people with mild Alzheimer's. They may substitute or make up words that sound like or mean something like the forgotten word. They sometimes even avoid talking to keep from making mistakes and appear subdued or withdrawn — especially in socially or mentally challenging situations.

They may also put things in very odd places. For example, a wallet may end up in the freezer, or clothes may go into the dishwasher. They may ask repetitive questions or hoard things of no value. When frustrated or tired, they may become uncharacteristically angry.

Common Changes in Mild AD:

- Loses spark or zest for life - does not start anything.
- Loses recent memory without a change in appearance or casual conversation.
- Loses judgment about money.
- Has difficulty with new learning and making new memories.
- Has trouble finding words - may substitute or make up words that sound like or mean something like the forgotten word.
- May stop talking to avoid making mistakes.
- Have shorter attention span and less motivation to stay with an activity.
- Easily loses way going to familiar places.
- Resists change or new things.
- Has trouble organizing and thinking logically.
- Asks repetitive questions.
- Withdraws, loses interest, and is irritable, not as sensitive to others' feelings, uncharacteristically angry when frustrated or tired.
- Will not make decisions. For example, when asked what she wants to eat, says "I'll have what she is having."
- Takes longer to do routine chores and becomes upset if rushed or if something unexpected happens.
- Forgets to pay, pays too much, or forgets how to pay - may hand the checkout person a wallet instead of the correct amount of money.
- Forgets to eat, eats only one kind of food, or eats constantly.
- Loses or misplaces things by hiding them in odd places or forgets where things go, such as putting clothes in the dishwasher.
- Constantly checks, searches or hoards things of no value.

```
┌─────────────────────────────────────────────────┐
│                  AD - Early                     │
│                                                 │
│  • Characteristics      • Interventions         │
│  • Begins with          • Medications - Aricept │
│    forgetfulness          and Cognex (both are  │
│  • Progresses to          commercial names)     │
│    disorientation and   • Therapy (deal with    │
│    confusion              depression that often │
│  • Personality changes    accompanies           │
│  • Symptoms of            diagnosis)            │
│    depression/manic     • Counseling with family│
│    behaviors                                    │
└─────────────────────────────────────────────────┘
```

You or your loved one might be experiencing some lapses in memory or other cognitive problems, but neither family nor friends are able to detect any changes. A medical exam would not reveal any problems either.

Family members and friends recognize mild changes in memory, communication patterns, or behavior. A visit to the doctor might result in a diagnosis of early-stage or mild Alzheimer's disease, but not always. Common symptoms in this stage include:

- Problems producing people's names or the right words for objects.
- Noticeable difficulty functioning in employment or social settings.
- Forgetting material that has just been read.
- Misplacing important objects with increasing frequency.
- Decrease in planning or organizational skills.

Cognitive decline is more evident. You or your loved one may become more forgetful of recent events or personal details. Other problems include impaired mathematical ability (for instance, difficulty counting backwards from 100 by 9s), a diminished ability to carry out complex tasks like throwing a party or managing finances, moodiness, and social withdrawal.

225

AD - Early

- Music Therapy
  - Used to relieve depression
  - Coupled with exercise and relaxation techniques
  - Increase or maintain social relationships (dancing, improvisation)
  - Maintain positive activities (church choir, handbell choir, senior social dances, etc. . .)

Music Therapy And Alzheimer's Disease
Source: (American Music Therapy Association, Inc.)

"...[W]e loses sight of how powerful melody and rhythm can be in the realm of medicine, particularly with respect to Alzheimer's patients and their caregivers... nursing homes and hospitals are finding that working with a music therapist can make a big difference..."

- C. Gorman. Time, November 14, 2005

What Is Music Therapy?
Music Therapy is the clinical and evidence-based use of music interventions to accomplish individualized goals within a therapeutic relationship by a credentialed professional who has completed an approved music therapy program. Music therapy interventions can be designed to promote wellness, manage stress, alleviate pain, enhance memory, improve communication, and provide unique opportunities for interaction. Research in music therapy supports the effectiveness of interventions in many areas such as facilitating movement and overall physical rehabilitation, increasing motivation to engage in treatment, providing emotional support for clients and their families, and creating an outlet for

expression of feelings. Because music therapy is a powerful and non-threatening medium, unique outcomes are possible.

How Does Music Therapy Make A Difference For Older Persons?

Music therapy treatment is efficacious and valid with older persons who have functional deficits in physical, psychological, cognitive, or social functioning. Research results and clinical experiences attest to the viability of music therapy even in those who are resistive to other treatment approaches. Music is a form of sensory stimulation, which provokes responses due to the familiarity, predictability, and feelings of security associated with it.

What Do Music Therapists Do?

After assessing the strengths and needs of each client, qualified music therapists develop a treatment plan with goals and objectives and then provide the indicated treatment. Music therapists structure the use of both instrumental and vocal music strategies to improve functioning or facilitate changes that contribute to life quality. They may improvise or compose music with clients, accompany and conduct group music experiences, provide instrument instruction, direct music and movement activities, or structure music listening opportunities. Music therapists are usually members of a health care interdisciplinary team and they implement programs with groups or individuals that display a vast continuum of needs, from leisure time classes and community involvement to bedside care.

Where Do Music Therapists Work?

Music therapists offer services in skilled and intermediate care facilities, adult foster care homes, rehabilitation hospitals, residential care facilities, hospitals, adult day care centers, retirement facilities, senior centers, hospices, senior evaluation programs, psychiatric treatment centers, and other facilities. Music therapists also work for agencies that provide in-home care. Some therapists are self-employed and provide individual and group music therapy services on a contract basis.

What Can One Expect From A Music Therapist?

When individualized music experiences are designed by a professionally trained music therapist to fit functional abilities and needs, responses may be immediate and readily apparent. Participants without a music background can benefit from music therapy.

Music therapy provides opportunities for:
- Memory recall which contributes to reminiscence and satisfaction with life.
- Positive changes in mood and emotional states.
- Sense of control over life through successful experiences.
- Awareness of self and environment which accompanies increased attention to music.
- Anxiety and stress reduction for older adult and caregiver.
- Nonpharmacological management of pain and discomfort.
- Stimulation which provokes interest even when no other approach is effective.
- Structure which promotes rhythmic and continuous movement or vocal fluency as an adjunct to physical rehabilitation.
- Emotional intimacy when spouses and families share creative music experiences.
- Social interaction with caregivers and families.

Who Is Qualified As A Music Therapist?

Graduates of colleges or universities from more than 70 approved music therapy programs are eligible to take a national examination administered by the Certification Board for Music Therapists (CBMT), an independent, non-profit certifying agency fully accredited by the National Commission for Certifying Agencies. After successful completion of the CBMT examination, graduates are issued the credential necessary for professional practice, Music Therapist-Board Certified (MT-BC). In addition to the MT-BC credential, other recognized professional designations are Registered Music Therapists (RMT), Certified Music Therapists (CMT), and Advanced Certified Music Therapist (ACMT) listed with the National Music Therapy Registry. Any individual who does not have proper training and credentials is not qualified to provide music therapy services.

How Does Music Therapy Help Families?
Music therapy provides:
- A forum to share common experiences and enjoyment as a couple or family.
- Meaningful time spent together in a positive, creative way.
- Relaxation for the entire family.
- Stimulation for reminiscence of family bonds.
- Unity and intimacy for families through verbal and nonverbal interaction.
- Respite for the caregiver.

Why Music Therapy?
The wife of a man with severe dementia said, "When I was encouraged by a music therapist to sing to my husband who had been lost in the fog of Alzheimer's disease for so many years, he looked at me and seemed to recognize me. On the last day of his life, he opened his eyes and looked into mine when I sang his favorite hymn. I will always treasure that last moment we shared together. Music therapy gave me that memory, the gift I will never forget."

Dr. Oliver Sacks, at the Hearing before the Senate Special Committee on Aging entitled, "Forever Young: Music and Aging," stated: "The power of music is very remarkable... One sees Parkinsonian patients unable to walk, but able to dance perfectly well or patients almost unable to talk, who are able to sing perfectly well... I think that music therapy and music therapists are crucial and indispensable in institutions for elderly people and among neurologically disabled patients."

A gentleman in the early stages of progressive dementia improvised on a xylophone during a music therapy session to express his feelings, and then stated: "I don't know how anyone can live without music."

A frail 93 year old woman, referred for music therapy after being diagnosed with major depression, said: "Now, there is no need to be morose. I can have my music here with me and listen to it whenever I want to feel young."

When a couple danced together for the first time after five years of the husband's deterioration from probable Alzheimer's disease, the wife said: "Thank you for helping us dance. It's the first time in three years that my husband held me in his arms." Tearfully, she said that she had missed him just holding her and that music therapy had made that possible.

Stage of AD - Moderate

- MMSE 11-20

- 3-6 years following diagnosis

- Aphasia and apraxia become more pronounced

- Loss of IADLS and increased assistance with ADLs

- Beginning to exhibit some neuropsych symptoms particularly paranoia

---

Moderate Alzheimer's Disease
Source: (National Institute on Aging)

In the middle stage of Alzheimer's, people cannot organize thoughts or follow logical explanations. They lose the ability to follow written instructions and often need help choosing proper clothing for the season or occasion. Eventually, they will require help getting dressed because their confusion may cause them to put their pajamas on over their daytime clothes or their shoes on the wrong feet. They may also have episodes of urinary or fecal incontinence.

It is usually during this stage that people start having problems recognizing family members and friends. They may mix up identities — thinking a son is a brother or that a spouse is a stranger. They may become confused about where they are and what day, season, or year it is. They become unable to recall their address or phone number.

Because they lack judgment and tend to wander, people with moderate Alzheimer's disease are not safe on their own. They may exhibit restless, repetitive movements in late afternoon, or continually repeat certain stories, words, or motions, such as tearing tissues.

Problems with communication worsen during the moderate stage of Alzheimer's. This can lead to a variety of challenging behaviors, including:

Paranoia that sometimes provokes accusations of infidelity or stealing

Agitation, frustration, or anger that can lead to cursing, kicking, hitting, biting, screaming, or grabbing

Common Changes in Moderate AD:
- Changes in behavior, concern for appearance, hygiene, and sleep become more noticeable.
- Mixes up identity of people, such as thinking a son is a brother or that a wife is a stranger.
- Poor judgment creates safety issues when left alone - may wander and risk exposure, poisoning, falls, self-neglect or exploitation.
- Has trouble recognizing familiar people and own objects; may take things that belong to others.
- Continuously repeats stories, favorite words, statements, or motions like tearing tissues.
- Have restless, repetitive movements in late afternoon or evening, such as pacing, trying doorknobs, fingering draperies.

- Cannot organize thoughts or follow logical explanations.
- Has trouble following written notes or completing tasks.
- Makes up stories to fill in gaps in memory. For example might say, "Mama will come for me when she gets off work."
- May be able to read but cannot formulate the correct response to a written request.
- May accuse, threaten, curse, fidget, or behave inappropriately, such as kicking, hitting, biting, screaming, or grabbing.
- May become sloppy or forget manners.
- May see, hear, smell, or taste things that are not there.
- May accuse spouse of an affair or family members of stealing.
- Naps frequently or awakens at night believing it is time to go to work.
- Has more difficulty positioning the body to use the toilet or sit in a chair.
- May think mirror image is following him or television story is happening to her.
- Needs help finding the toilet, using the shower, remembering to drink, and dressing for the weather or occasion.
- Exhibits inappropriate sexual behavior, such as mistaking another individual for a spouse. Forgets what private behavior is, and may disrobe or masturbate in public.

AD - Middle

- **Characteristics**
- Need assistance with ADLs
- Unable to remember names
- Loss of short-term recall
- May display anxious, agitated, delusional, or obsessive behavior
- May be physically or verbally aggressive

- Poor personal hygiene
- Disturbed sleep
- Inability to carry on a conversation
- May use "word salad" (sentence fragments)
- Posture may be altered
- Disoriented to time and place
- May ask questions repeatedly

Some assistance with daily tasks is required. Problems with memory and thinking are quite noticeable, including symptoms such as:

- An inability to recall one's own contact information or key details about one's history.
- Disorientation to time and/or place.
- Decreased judgment and skills in regard to personal care.

Even though symptoms are worsening, people in this stage usually still know their own name and the names of key family members and can eat and use the bathroom without assistance.

This is often the most difficult stage for caregivers because it is characterized by personality and behavior changes. In addition, memory continues to decline, and assistance is required for most daily activities. The most common symptoms associated with this stage include:

- Reduced awareness of one's surroundings and of recent events.
- Problems recognizing one's spouse and other close family members, although faces are still distinguished between familiar and unfamiliar.

- Sundowning, which is increased restlessness and agitation in the late afternoon and evening.
- Difficulty using the bathroom independently.
- Bowel and bladder incontinence.
- Suspicion.
- Repetitive behavior (verbal and/or nonverbal).
- Wandering.

AD - Middle

- **Interventions**
- Validation Therapy
- Structured Areas for Mobility
- Positive, nurturing, loving environment

- Music Therapy
- Provides avenue for social interaction (Instrumental Improvisation; TGS, Guided Music Listening)
- Provides a medium for verbal/non-verbal expression (TGS)
- Can help maintain cognitive and affective functioning

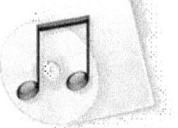

Designs for Validation Therapy
Source: (CBS Interactive Business Netword, Mark Warner, 2000)

This technique can be supported in the Alzheimer's environment

As each member of the group sat in the circle hoping the balloon would gently drift their way, Roxanne burst from her chair in a fit of rage, shouting "There'll be no ball-playing in my house!"
Furious at the insolence of the players who ignored her commands, Roxanne forcefully attacked a staff member, who tried to comfort her by explaining that she was not in her house, but merely with her friends playing a game. Roxanne did not buy that and swung wildly, hitting the staff member squarely in the chest.

Fearing that I, too, might fall victim to the same fate, I cautiously approached Roxanne. I put my arm around her shoulder and supported her in her cause that there should be no ball-playing in her house. "This is terrible," I said. "You're right, they should not be throwing that ball in your house, should they?"

"No, they shouldn't," bellowed Roxanne, showing only the slightest relief that someone saw her point of view.

"But you know, Roxanne, the only way they will stop throwing that ball is if we write down the rules for them. I think it's the only way they'll listen." Roxanne was buying this approach, so I suggested, "Let's go into that room over there and write down all the rules for them, okay?" Much to my relief, Roxanne agreed and hand-in-hand we went into the room to write down the "rules."

"Okay," I began, "Rule Number One is 'No ball-playing in the house,' right?"

"That's right," agreed Roxanne.

"So what will Rule Number Two be," I asked, and then offered, "How about, 'No running in the house'?"

"That's right," said Roxanne, "my grandchildren are not allowed to run in my house."

"Roxanne, you've got grandchildren," I said, raising the tone of my voice with delight.

"Oh, yes, my little growing boy is six years old, and he is as smart as they come." Roxanne was on a roll now, and the upset caused earlier by the balloon toss in the next room might as well have been miles away. Fifteen minutes later, when the game was over, Roxanne and I emerged from the room, both of us just as happy as we could be, the "rules" left on the table and the incident long forgotten.

The technique used here is called Validation Therapy. It assumes that no matter what illusion the person with Alzheimer's disease (AD) is living, she is right, and nothing you can say or do will convince her otherwise. Naomi Feil is the acknowledged expert on validation therapy and wrote the book The Validation Breakthrough. The basic concept is that you have to buy into the resident's illusion and convincingly play along with it, there by validating it. Eventually you will see opportunities to mold the tale--and the resident's behavior--into something that is acceptable and no longer upsetting.

"What has this got to do with design," you ask? Everything, in fact. Understanding Alzheimer's disease and the many creative ways to deal with it are as much a challenge of designing an environment as of caregiving within it.

Angie is always complaining about the stranger in the bathroom. She will not use the toilet while "the other lady" is in there. She says that the bathroom is occupied, not realizing it is her own reflection that she sees. Do you explain that she is seeing herself in a mirror?

No. You go along with her. How about, "I'm sorry, Angie, let me see what's taking that lady so long." You go into the bathroom and somehow cover the mirror. One family confronted by this situation told their mother that the mirror was dirty and needed to be cleaned. They sprayed it with a powdered deodorant, creating a haze that obscured any reflection. "Mom, she's out of there now," her daughter said. "I wonder what took her so long. Let me know if you need anything. I'll be right here waiting for you."

Caregiver 1: "Deborah won't eat anything. She just sits at the table and stares at the food. She loves gardening, though; we spend hours every day weeding and pruning the vegetables in our garden."

A golden opportunity awaits us here. Figure it out. Deborah loves gardening, but will not eat.

"So we tried something a little different. Though the tomatoes were days from ripening, I went to the grocery store and picked out some beautiful red ones. Instead of putting them on the table in front of her, I pretended to come in from the garden, tomatoes in hand. As Deborah Looked at the tomatoes, I told her, 'They came from our garden, and don't they look delicious?'"

Granted, such ploys are not always so successful, but many are. Sharing the bounty of the garden, enjoying the fruits of your labor that you grew together, can somehow trigger pleasant, guiding thoughts and behaviors when all else fails. Perhaps it stirs up memories from long ago, or maybe it is just the thrill of eating your own garden vegetables. Regardless, it adds a new dimension to life that might very well conquer the ravages of the disease and perhaps bring new purpose to those waist-high gardens many facilities are installing these days.

Taking validation to the next step often involves anticipating the problem and creating the illusion. Validation also referred to as deceptive therapy, white lies and fiblets, means creating a story--in the best interest of the person who is "confused."

"Dad, who's president? Do you remember his name?"

"Of course l do, it's Roosevelt!"

If your family member believes it is the 1930s, so be it. As he regresses in time, so do his memories of values, experiences and people. What was important then becomes important now!

Given residents' belief that they are living when Roosevelt was president, what would the world have been like back then? What would the good experiences and environmental features have been? How can we recreate the familiar feelings of that period in a convincing and subtle way?

For example, those were the days when they hung the clothes on a line in the back yard. Isn't that the kind of good and secure feeling we would want to recreate--possibly by merely providing a clothesline? Others might be enjoying the time when they were raising their families. What better way to indulge them than by allowing them to once again care for their spouse or children by hanging "their" clothes out to dry?

Or, perhaps they have less comforting memories.

Caregiver 2: "Mom collects everything--rubber bands, paper clips paper...everything! And she stores them everywhere. You can hardly walk in her room, there is so much stuff in there!"

Perhaps Mom is reliving times when the country was at war, when every little scrap was valuable in the war effort, or the Great Depression, when times were so tough that you had to keep everything, when nothing that might be useful was thrown out. Environmental validation then might mean providing easy-to-see drawers, trunks, or cabinets to store these important items.

How were evenings spent in the good old days (before TV, let us say)? Many families spent hours sitting on the porch, watching people go by, talking to neighbors, etc. Why not create a porch, complete with rockers and swing gliders? Locate it carefully and safely, but within view of interesting activities (maybe a playground where children play). Make sure it is secure for those who might try to leave or climb over the railing; it should also be far enough from strangers outside who might be perceived as intruding into their space. Perhaps a screened porch would do the trick.

One should also beware of environmental miscues.

"Bruce, why aren't you eating?"

"I didn't bring my wallet and can't pay for the meal."

Although Bruce is living in an assisted living facility and does not have to pay for his meal, he does not realize that. As far as he is concerned, this large, beautiful dining room is a restaurant, and the more he eats, the bigger the bill. Perhaps if we had divided the room into smaller, more homelike dining rooms and spared the expense of the huge chandelier, Bruce would feel more comfortable with his home-cooked meal.

Do not forget that little environmental touches can mean a lot.

Caregiver 3: "My mother refused to take a bath. For years, soaking in a warm tub of water had been the highlight of her day. But now, for some reason, she feared the tub and everything it represented. Eventually she confided in me, relating a childhood story about a little girl who got sucked down the bathtub drain. She recalled that tale and, like that little girl, she was afraid that she too might fall victim to that terrible fate. The solution: We put a mat over the drain. Her fear suddenly disappeared."

In a daycare center, angry and impatient residents wait for their rides to take them home. Each time the door opens, one, two, or even three of them race to it and powerfully attempt to get into the van, which has actually arrived to transport someone else. Staffs members intervene, often unsuccessfully, overcome by the strength and determination of people with a very important cause (the van is there for them). If we, as facility planners and designers, can anticipate this kind of behavior, we can plan door placement to eliminate visibility of the van outside, thus avoiding this upsetting and potentially volatile situation. There are design solutions for problems like these, if problems are simply acknowledged and thought about ahead of time.

Although the stories I have recounted are all too familiar to healthcare professionals, they are often "Greek" to design professionals. Nevertheless, it is a design credo: To design for any client, you have to understand the client. Why should those who have Alzheimer's disease be treated any differently?

We are only in the earliest days of learning how to design for dementia. Hopefully, there will soon be a cure for these devastating diseases, making an article such as this a moot exercise. But until then, we must continue to delve into our creative minds, take chances, and discover what works and what does not for this population. Nursing home/assisted living managers should help designers understand how people with dementia perceive and interpret their worlds. Only when equipped with this knowledge can we designers begin to address these problems with the tools that we have available to us.

AD Stage - Severe

- Usually 6-10 years following diagnosis
- Severe language disturbances: mutism, echolalia, repetitive vocalizations
- Pronounced neuropsych manifestations including agitation, aggression
- Very late in course can see muscle rigidity, gait disturbances, incontinence, dysphagia

---

Severe Alzheimer's Disease
People in the last stage of Alzheimer's require help with all their daily needs. They lose the ability to walk without assistance and then the ability to sit up without support. They are usually incontinent and may no longer speak coherently. They rarely recognize family members. Swallowing difficulties can cause choking, and they may refuse to eat.

AD - Late

- **Characteristics**
- Loss of verbal articulation
- Loss of ambulation
- Bowel and bladder incontinence
- Extended sleep patterns
- Unresponsive to most stimuli

- **Interventions**
- Caring for physical needs
- Medical interventions
- Most activities are inaccessible

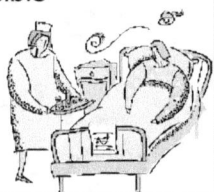

In the final stage, it is usually no longer possible to respond to the surrounding environment. You or your loved one may be able to speak words or short phrases, but communication is extremely limited. Basic functions begin to shut down, such as motor coordination and the ability to swallow. Total care is required around the clock.

Although the stages provide a blueprint for the progression of Alzheimer's symptoms, not everyone advances through the stages similarly. Caregivers report that their loved ones sometimes seem to be in two or more stages at once, and the rate at which people advance through the stages is highly individual. Still, the stages help us understand Alzheimer's symptoms and prepare for their accompanying challenges.

Common Changes in Severe AD:
Source: (National Institute on Aging)
- Does not recognize self or close family.
- Speaks in gibberish, is mute, or is difficult to understand.
- May refuse to eat, chokes, or forgets to swallow.
- May repetitively cry out, pat, or touch everything.
- Loses control of bowel and bladder.

- Loses weight and skin becomes thin and tears easily.
- May look uncomfortable or cry out when transferred or touched.
- Forgets how to walk or is too unsteady or weak to stand alone.
- May have seizures, frequent infections, falls.
- May groan, scream, or mumble loudly.
- Sleeps more.
- Needs total assistance for all activities of daily living.

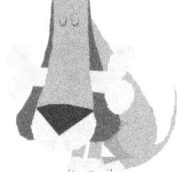

AD - Late

- **Music Therapy**
  - Tape by bedside
  - Gentle singing by therapist ~ one-sided, client will not participate
  - Can provide some connection between patient and family members through singing
  - Use a calm voice
  - Utilize touch: holding hands, hugging, rocking, hand on shoulder, etc. . .

- **Art Therapy**

- **Pet Therapy**

Music, Art, and Other Therapies
Source: (Alzheimer's Association)

Introduction
Music, art, pet, and other types of therapies can help enrich the lives of people with Alzheimer's disease. Pets, for instance, have been shown to reduce depression and boost self-esteem. Art provides an outlet for expression. Music stirs memories, emotions and when accompanied by singing, encourages group activity.

Music Therapy
- Identify music that is familiar and enjoyable to the listeners.
- Use live music, tapes, or CDs; radio programs, interrupted by too many commercials, can cause confusion.
- Use music to create the mood you want.
- Link music with other reminiscence activities; use photographs to help stir memories.
- Encourage movement (clapping, dancing) to add to the enjoyment.
- Avoid sensory overload; eliminate competing noises by shutting windows and doors and by turning off the television.

Art Therapy
- Keep the project on an adult level. Avoid anything that might be demeaning or seem child-like.
- Build conversation into the project. Provide encouragement, discuss what the person is creating, and try to initiate a bit of creative storytelling or reminiscence.
- Help the person begin the activity. If the person is painting, you may need to start the brush movement. Most other projects should only require basic instruction and assistance.
- Use safe materials. Avoid toxic substances and sharp tools.
- Allow plenty of time to complete the art project.
- The person does not have to finish the project in one sitting.
- And remember: The artwork is complete when the person says it is.

Pet Therapy Guidelines :
- Not everyone will react positively to animals. Those who owned pets previously tend to be more responsive.
- Match the animal's activity and energy level with that of the individual. For example, a lively dog might be appropriate for someone who can go out for a walk; a cat may be more appropriate for a person who is less mobile.

- For more information about alternative therapies, contact your local Alzheimer's Association or refer to the resource list provided by the Alzheimer's Association's Green-Field Library.

III. C. AD and Dementia Behavior

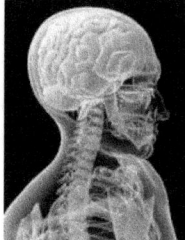

Dr. Jerry Turner
IEP, Inc.

www.RCFE-CEU.com

This next section is applicable to Dementia and non-Dementia clients. For the purpose of this course we will focus on dementia clients. However, rules of behavior are basic and apply, to one degree or another, to all behaviors. Certain exceptions are noted and discussed. The effects of dementia will play a critical role on behavior, but not on understanding the behavior. The basic goal of psychology applies to behavior – If you can observe a behavior, you can describe a behavior, and if you can explain the behavior you can predict and control the behavior.

Many of you may use these principals in behavior modification; others may simply seek a better understanding of behaviors.

Behavior Types

- Wandering
- Finding a missing client
- Protecting the patient
- Belligerence, anger or aggressive behavior
- Hallucinations, illusions or paranoia
- Sleep problems
- Eating difficulties

Alzheimer's Behavior Management
Source: (HelpGuide.org)

Learn to Manage Common Behavior Problems
The confusion and disorientation of mid-stage Alzheimer's bring increasing difficulty with maintaining normal behaviors. The result may be inappropriate behavior in social situations or getting lost in one's own house. Alzheimer's patients can become a danger to themselves or others.

Alzheimer's patients may have a wide variety of behavioral problems including wandering; rummaging through or hiding things; aggressiveness; hallucinations or paranoia; and sleeping and eating problems.

Most behavior problems pose serious difficulties for the person trying to provide care. Management of this behavior will require the caregiver to modify the home environment and change communication styles.

Management of Wandering
Wandering around the house may be irritating to the caregiver, but not necessarily unsafe for the client. In this case, you may need to

adjust your anxiety level about wandering. On the other hand, some wandering can be dangerous and must be prevented: going into areas of the house that are off-limits, especially stairwells, decks, hot tubs, and swimming pools; leaving the house alone via a window or door to go outside; or leaving your yard or property.

You can prevent many instances of wandering by carefully selecting child-safety devices for your home that effectively restrict adults. Some caregivers have "outsmarted" the person who has a desire to escape with novel solutions, such as hiding items like purses, shoes, or glasses that the person would always take with them if they left the house. Or, you may want to acquire comfortable chairs that are difficult for the Alzheimer's client to get out of! Bean bag chairs and recliners are pleasant to sit in, yet restrict movement out of the chair.

Two characteristic precursors to wandering are restlessness and disorientation. Redirecting behaviors, distracting, orienting, and encouraging physical exercise therefore, serve to reduce the incidence of wandering. Some suggestions are:

- **Immediately redirect pacing or restless behavior into productive activity** or purposeful exercise.
- **Make sure the Alzheimer's client gets plenty of exercise** and movement. Even consider singing and dancing! Indoor shopping malls are vast walking opportunities protected from the weather. If you walk outdoors, make sure that you and the client have clothing that shelters from cold, rain, and sun.
- **Make sure the person is involved in many productive daily activities**, such as the simple chores of folding laundry or washing vegetables for dinner.
- **Reassure the person if they appear disoriented.**
- **If wandering tends to occur at a particular time of day, distract the person at that time.**
- **Reduce noise levels and confusion.** These can disorient the person.
- **Disorientation can be a result of medication side-effects, drug interactions, or over-medicating.** If disorientation

is becoming a problem, consult the doctor.

If you are moving the client to a new environment, **reduce disorientation by acclimating them** ahead of time with several visits.

Planning for When the Alzheimer's Client does Wander

In case an Alzheimer's client in your care *does* wander, it is a good idea to have a plan in place. Make a list of what you should do if the person becomes lost – include telephone numbers to call, places to check, etc. Notify neighbors and local police about your Alzheimer's client's tendency to wander, and ask them to call you if they see your elder wandering without supervision.

If a police search becomes necessary, you will need a recent photo of the person's face. You can make the searchers' jobs easier by also having a video of the person to be able to show them, and by keeping on hand some unwashed clothing from the elder to help search-and-rescue dogs. (To do this properly, place the clothing in a plastic bag with plastic-gloved hands, and replace this clothing monthly.) Another smart preventative measure is to sign up the client for the Alzheimer's Association's Safe Return Program, which is an identification system to help rescue lost Alzheimer's patients who have wandered away.

Where to Look for a Lost Alzheimer's Client

Rescue is urgent for a wandering person who has Alzheimer's or another dementia. The person may not call out for help or answer your calls. And people in this situation often do not leave many physical cues. The person may get stuck in a place that they cannot get out of, and he or she can die from exposure if left outside too long. Dehydration and hypothermia are dangers. Some ideas about where to find the wanderer:

Finding a Missing Alzheimer's Client
- **Check dangerous areas** near the home, such as bodies of water, open stairwells, dense foliage, tunnels, bus stops, high balconies, and heavily traveled roads.
- **Look within a one-mile radius** of where the client was before they wandered.

- **Look within one hundred feet of a road**, as most wanderers start out on roads and remain close by. Especially look carefully into bushes and ditches, as the person may have fallen or gotten caught.
- **Search in the direction of the wanderer's dominant hand**. People usually travel first in their dominant direction.
- **Investigate familiar places**, such as former residences or favorite spots. Often, wandering has a particular destination.
- **If you suspect that the person used a car or public transportation** to go away, you must think of likely places to search that are farther away.

Management of Rummaging Around or Hiding Things

Caring for a client who rummages around or hides things in the home is a challenge, but not an insurmountable one.

Protecting your Property

Lock certain rooms or cabinets to protect their contents, and lock up all valuables. Have mail delivered out of reach of the Alzheimer's client--perhaps to a post office box. If items do disappear, learn the person has preferred hiding places and look there first to find hidden objects. Restrict access to wastebaskets and trashcans, and check all wastebaskets before disposing of their contents, in case objects have been hidden there.

Protecting Alzheimer's Patients from Harming Themselves

Remove or prevent access to unsafe substances, such as cleaning products, alcohol, and medications. Patients with dementia sometimes overdose on alcohol. Prevent electrical accidents by blocking unused electrical outlets with childproofing devices. It may also be helpful to designate a special drawer of items that the person can safely "play" with when they are bored.

Management of Belligerence, Anger, or Aggressive Behavior

Following are some ideas about caring for an aggressive Alzheimer's client. Consider each idea independently of the others.

- **Do not confront the person or try to discuss the angry behavior.** The person with dementia cannot reflect on their unacceptable behavior and cannot learn to control it.
- **Do not initiate physical contact during the angry outburst.** Often, physical contact triggers physical violence in the client.
- **Provide the person with a "time-out" away from you.** Let them have space to be angry by themselves. Withdraw in the direction of a safe exit.
- **Distract the person to a more pleasurable topic or activity.**
- **Look for patterns in the aggression.** Consider factors such as privacy, independence, boredom, pain, or fatigue. Avoid those activities or topics that anger the person. To help find any patterns, you might keep a log of when the aggressive episodes occur.
  If the person gets angry when tasks are too difficult for them, **break down tasks into smaller pieces.**
- **Minimize stress and novelty.**
- **Maintain calm within yourself.** Getting anxious or upset in response may escalate the aggressiveness.
- **Let the person play out the aggression.** Just be sure that you are safe and that they are safe themselves.
- **Get help from others** during the activities that anger the client.
- **Do not take the aggressiveness personally.**

Management of Hallucinations, Illusions, or Paranoia
Hallucinations can be the result of failing senses. Unidentifiable sounds, shadows, and highly contrasting colors all can become the basis for fantasy. Decrease the number of things in the environment that can be misinterpreted as something else, such as patterned wallpaper or bright, contrasting surfaces or objects. Increase lighting so that there are few shadows while avoiding glare, and remove or cover mirrors if they cause problems. Maintaining sameness in the environment may also help reduce hallucinations. Also, violent movies or television can contribute to paranoia – avoid letting the client watch disturbing programs.

When hallucinations or illusions do occur, do not argue about what is real and what is fantasy. Discuss the client's feelings relative to what they imagine they see. Respond to the emotional content of what the person is saying, rather than to the factual/fictional content.

Medications can sometimes help to reduce hallucinations, so seek professional advice if you are concerned about this problem.

Management of Nighttime Wakefulness and Other Sleep Problems

Brain disease often disrupts the sleep-wake cycle. Alzheimer's patients may have wakefulness, disorientation, and confusion beginning at dusk and continuing throughout the night. This is called "sundowning." There are two aspects to sundowning. First, confusion, over-stimulation, and fatigue during the day may result in increased confusion, restlessness, and insecurity at night. And second, some Alzheimer's patients have fear of the dark, perhaps because of the lack of familiar daytime noises and activity. The client may seek out security and protection at night to alleviate their discomfort.

Following are some strategies to reduce nighttime restlessness:

Improve Sleep Hygiene

Physical activities will help the person feel more tired at bedtime. Walk with the person during the day. If the person seems very fatigued during the day, give them a short rest in the afternoon to regain their composure. This can lead to a better night's sleep. But do not let them sleep too long – too much daytime napping can increase nighttime wakefulness. Also, limit the client's caffeine intake.

Be consistent with the time for sleeping, and keep a routine for getting ready for bed.

Create a Calm Atmosphere for Sleeping

Give the person a bath and some warm milk before bed. Provide a comfortable bed, reduce noise and light, and play soothing music to help them get to sleep.

Close the curtains and leave a night light on all night. Some people with dementia imagine things in the dark and become upset. Stuffed animals or a pet may soothe the client and allow them to sleep.

Have the person use the toilet right before bedtime. Place a commode next to the bed for nighttime urination. Walking to the bathroom in the middle of the night may wake the person up too much, and then they cannot get back to sleep. The person may prefer to sleep in a chair or on the couch, rather than in bed. Furniture must be designed so that the client will not fall out while sleeping.

Resolve Common Problems
If the client paces during the night, make sure that the primary daytime caregiver can sleep. This requires either a very safe room for the client to pace in, or else another caregiver who takes over at night. You need your rest, too. Do not restrain the client in bed, but consider a hospital bed with guard rails in the later stages of Alzheimer's.
If night wakefulness has gotten too hard for you to manage, consult with a doctor if you wish to try administering sleeping pills.

Management of Refusing to Eat
Try any of or a combination of the following suggestions to care for a client who will not eat:
- **Encourage some exercise.** Exercise can make a person feel hungrier: The hungrier the person feels, the more likely they are to eat.
- **Monitor medications** some medications interfere with appetite. Read about the side effects of any medications that the Alzheimer's client is taking. Discuss with the doctor the lack of interest in eating; you may need to change a medication. Make sure that the person gets enough liquids with their food, as dry mouth may be a side-effect of some medications.
- **Make mealtimes pleasing to the client** if the Alzheimer's client does not like the person who is feeding them, they

may not feel like eating. Try a different caretaker for the feeding process. Make the client's favorite food, and serve food on colored tableware - dishes that contrast highly with food colors. Reduce distractions in the eating area. Also, avoid foods that are too hot or too cold, as these may be unpleasant to the client.

- **Feed the client like a baby** Try giving the client little spoonful's, and sing short, funny rhymes to get them to eat. Get the person to smile so that the mouth opens, and then slip a little food in their mouth. Or put a bit of the food on the person's lips so that they open their mouth wider. Provide finger foods and children's sipper cups: The person may have trouble using utensils and normal cups.

- **Monitor chewing and swallowing** Chewing and swallowing difficulties can develop as Alzheimer's progresses. If necessary, give instructions on when to chew and when to swallow. Keep the person upright for thirty minutes after eating so that they do not choke.

- **Transition into providing only puréed or soft foods** in the later stages of Alzheimer's, the person can no longer swallow food and may choke on food. Swallowing problems can lead to pneumonia because the client may inhale food or liquid into the lungs. Begin feeding only liquids to the client when the time is right - In the later stages of Alzheimer's, the person can no longer process solid foods.

At the end stage of Alzheimer's or another terminal illness, the client's organ systems begin to shut down and the lack of desire to eat or drink is the usual result. In the final days or hours, starvation or dehydration are not a problem and not a cause of suffering.

Understanding Behaviors

- Why do we do what we do?
  - Freud – Seek pleasure, avoid pain
  - Behaviorist – Conditioning

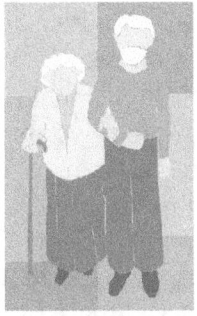

The Pain and Pleasure Principle
Source: (World Village, 2010)

The pain and pleasure principle, also known as the pleasure principal, is universal. It guides us in virtually everything we do, whether we are aware of it or not. Simply put, the pleasure principle states that people are driven to seek pleasure and to avoid pain. In other words, we are willing to do things that will bring us pleasure and we are unwilling to do things that will cause us pain.

It seems however that the two forces are out of balance. The avoidance of pain often wins from the desire to seek pleasure. Perhaps in the case of physical pain this seems logical, at least to a certain extent. But in most cases we are not talking about physical pain. Most often people choose to do things, or rather not to do certain things, in order to avoid emotional pain. Some people go even further and simply state that people avoid pain, they do not seek pleasure. People may know very well that in order to achieve certain results they desire, something needs to be done. They may even have a high degree of certainty that doing that something will indeed produce the desired result. But if that something makes them feel bad or even slightly uncomfortable, they are out. Of course logically this does not make any sense. Rationally we know

253

that we can get to C is we just put A and B together. But the fact is: we are not as rational as we sometimes claim to be. Human beings are mainly emotional creatures. We take decisions emotionally and then we try to back them up with logic.

The pain and pleasure principle, also known as the pleasure principal, is universal. It guides us in virtually everything we do, whether we are aware of it or not. Simply put, the pleasure principle states that people are driven to seek pleasure and to avoid pain. In other words, we are willing to do things that will bring us pleasure and we are unwilling to do things that will cause us pain. Sounds pretty obvious doesn't it?

It seems however that the two forces are out of balance. The avoidance of pain often wins from the desire to seek pleasure. Perhaps in the case of physical pain this seems logical, at least to a certain extent. But in most cases we're not talking about physical pain. Most often people choose to do things, or rather not to do certain things, in order to avoid emotional pain. Some people go even further and simply state that people avoid pain, they do not seek pleasure. People may know very well that in order to achieve certain results they desire, something needs to be done. They may even have a high degree of certainty that doing that something will indeed produce the desired result. But if that something makes them feel bad or even slightly uncomfortable, they are out. Of course logically this does not make any sense. Rationally we know that we can get to C is we just put A and B together. But the fact is: we are not as rational as we sometimes claim to be. Human beings are mainly emotional creatures. We take decisions emotionally and then we try to back them up with logic.

Most people would agree that the drive to avoid pain is stronger than the drive to seek pleasure. One of the reasons why this drive is this strong is because it is built into our biological survival system. Physical pain will cause people to automatically withdraw from what they perceive to be the source of their pain. Rationally we know that physical and emotional pain are not the same, but since the human brain has difficulty distinguishing real pain from perceived pain, most people react to it in exactly the same way.

"So why is this relevant for my business? You might say. Well, first of all if this is true for most people, it is probably true for you too. You may not realize it, but you have probably fallen into this trap more than once. More importantly; if you remain unaware of this, you will continue to do so. And regardless of what business you are in, that will hurt your bottom line. If you are in a business where you are dealing with other people, you should be aware that they are subject to the same exact principle. As a network marketer you are dealing almost exclusively with people. Therefore understanding this principle and applying it will prove to be crucial to your business success. Some of you may be using it without even knowing it. If you have a successful upline that teaches you exactly what to do and what to say there is a good chance that this principle is, at least partially, embedded into their training systems.

Many times we try to move people into action by getting them to focus on the pleasure they can get when they reach success. Although this can be very successful, there are many times when your prospect just does not seem to get excited about the potential rewards. You may have banged your head against the wall a couple of times. Perhaps you have mentally labeled your prospect as one of those poor unfortunate folks that just do not get it. People that are not the least bit interested in improving the quality of their life. Granted, over time you probably will run into a couple of those, but the majority of people you meet will not fall into that category. Most people really do want a better quality of life; they want more free time, more money, more respect, and more success. What is holding them back is fear. They fear change and associate pain with taking the necessary actions to make it happen. Obviously they perceive taking action as more painful than staying where they are at right now. And thus, they choose not to take the necessary actions.

In order to successfully move people into action you will have to apply the pain and pleasure principle on at least two levels. First you must apply it on yourself. Look closely at the way you conduct your business and you will inevitably find that there are many things you should do or do differently. You know you should be prospecting, presenting, and duplicating and you also know that you have to be strong to lead your people. But why aren't you? Simple answer: you associate pain with either one of those steps. In order to change this it will help if you start associating pain with not doing all those things. Think of how it will hurt you in the long run if you continue not taking action. You will find that when the pain of not doing it gets worse than the pain of doing it, you will decide to do whatever it is that needs to be done.

The second step is to apply this principle on your people. If you do this successfully you will find that you can actually make fear work for you. To illustrate this, picture yourself in a face to face encounter with a wild - and hungry - animal, for example a lion. If it is in front of you and you continue facing it, chances are the fear will paralyze you. And if you are fortunate enough to come to your senses before the lion gets to you, one thing is certain: moving forward will be the last thing on your mind. You can only move backwards and we all know how fast that goes. Instead, if you were to turn around and get the object of your fear behind you, you would discover just how fast you really can be. You would probably have little problems with some of the hurdles along your escape. In fact you would give many professional athletes a run for their money.

Conditioning
Source: (Wikipedia, 2010)

Classical Conditioning (also Pavlovian or Respondent Conditioning) is a form of associative learning that was firstly demonstrated by Ivan Pavlov. The typical procedure for inducing classical conditioning involves presentations of a neutral stimulus along with a stimulus of some significance. The neutral stimulus could be any event that does not result in an overt behavioral response from the organism under investigation. Pavlov referred to this as a Conditioned Stimulus (CS). Conversely, presentation of the significant stimulus necessarily evokes an innate, often reflexive, response. Pavlov called these the Unconditioned Stimulus (US) and Unconditioned Response (UR), respectively. If the CS and the US are repeatedly paired, eventually the two stimuli become associated and the organism begins to produce a behavioral response to the CS. Pavlov called this the Conditioned Response (CR).

Theories of Classical Conditioning
There are two competing theories of how classical conditioning works. The first, stimulus-response theory, suggests that an association to the unconditioned stimulus is made with the conditioned stimulus within the brain, but without involving conscious thought. The second theory stimulus-stimulus theory involves cognitive activity, in which the conditioned stimulus is associated to the concept of the unconditioned stimulus, a subtle but important distinction.

Stimulus-response theory, referred to as S-R theory, is a theoretical model of behavioral psychology that suggests humans and other animals can learn to associate a new stimulus- the conditioned stimulus (CS)- with a pre-existing stimulus - the unconditioned stimulus (US), and can think, feel or respond to the CS as if it were actually the US.

The opposing theory, put forward by cognitive behaviorists, is stimulus-stimulus theory (S-S theory). Stimulus-stimulus theory, referred to as S-S theory, is a theoretical model of classical conditioning that suggests a cognitive component is required to understand classical conditioning and that stimulus-response theory is an inadequate model. It proposes that a cognitive component is at play. S-R theory suggests that an animal can learn to associate a conditioned stimulus (CS) such as a bell, with the impending arrival of food termed the unconditioned stimulus, resulting in an observable behavior such as salivation. Stimulus-stimulus theory suggests that instead the animal salivates to the bell because it is associated with the concept of food, which is a very fine but important distinction.

To test this theory, psychologist Robert Rescorla undertook the following experiment. Rats learned to associate a loud noise as the unconditioned stimulus, and a light as the conditioned stimulus.

The response of the rats was to freeze and cease movement. What would happen then if the rats were habituated to the US? S-R theory would suggest that the rats would continue to respond to the US, but if S-S theory is correct, they would be habituated to the concept of a loud sound (danger), and so would not freeze to the CS. The experimental results suggest that S-S was correct, as the rats no longer froze when exposed to the signal light. His theory still continues and is applied in everyday life.

Understanding Behaviors

- Why do we do what we do?

  - Humanistic – Self-actualization
  - Evolutionist – Beneficial for survival & procreation
  - Biologist – Homeostasis

The Humanistic View of Human Behavior
Source: (Asociation for Humanistic Psychology)

Humanistic psychology is a value orientation that holds a hopeful, constructive view of human beings and of their substantial capacity to be self-determining. It is guided by a conviction that intentionality and ethical values are strong psychological forces, among the basic determinants of human behavior. This conviction leads to an effort to enhance such distinctly human qualities as choice, creativity, the interaction of the body, mind and spirit, and the capacity to become more aware, free, responsible, life-affirming, and trustworthy.

Humanistic psychology acknowledges that the mind is strongly influenced by determining forces in society and in the unconscious, and that some of these are negative and destructive. Humanistic psychology nevertheless emphasizes the independent dignity and worth of human beings and their conscious capacity to develop personal competence and self-respect. This value orientation has led to the development of therapies to facilitate personal and interpersonal skills and to enhance the quality of life.

Since there is much difficulty involved in inner growth, humanistic psychologists often stress the importance of courageously learning to take responsibility for oneself as one confronts personal transitions. The difficulty of encouraging personal growth is matched by the difficulty of developing appropriate institutional and organizational environments in which human beings can flourish. Clearly, societies both help and hinder human growth. Because nourishing environments can make an important contribution to the development of healthy personalities, human needs should be given priority when fashioning social policies. ,This becomes increasingly critical in a rapidly changing world threatened by such dangers as nuclear war, overpopulation and the breakdown of traditional social structures.

Many humanistic psychologists stress the importance of social change, the challenge of modifying old institutions and inventing new ones able to sustain both human development and organizational efficacy. Thus the humanistic emphasis on individual freedom should be matched by recognition of our interdependence and our responsibilities to one another, to society and culture, and to the future.

Evolutionist
Evolutionary psychology (EP) attempts to explain mental and psychological traits—such as memory, perception, or language— as adaptations, that is, as the functional products of natural selection or sexual selection. Adaptationist thinking about physiological mechanisms, such as the heart, lungs, and immune system, is common in evolutionary biology. Evolutionary psychology applies the same thinking to psychology.

Evolutionary psychologists (see, for example, Buss, 2005; Durrant & Ellis, 2003; Pinker, 2002; Tooby & Cosmides, 2005) argue that much of human behavior is generated by psychological adaptations that evolved to solve recurrent problems in human ancestral environments. They hypothesize, for example, that humans have inherited special mental capacities for acquiring language, making it nearly automatic, while inheriting no capacity specifically for reading and writing. Other adaptations, according to EP, might include the abilities to infer others' emotions, to discern kin from non-kin, to identify and prefer healthier mates, to cooperate with others, and so on. Consistent with the theory of natural selection, evolutionary psychology sees organisms as often in conflict with others of their species, including mates and relatives. For example, mother mammals and their young offspring sometimes struggle over weaning, which benefits the mother more than the child. Humans, however, have a marked capacity for cooperation under certain conditions as well.

Evolutionary psychologists see those behaviors and emotions that are nearly universal, such as fear of spiders and snakes, as more likely to reflect evolved adaptations. Evolved psychological adaptations (such as the ability to learn a language) interact with cultural inputs to produce specific behaviors (e.g., the specific language learned). This view is contrary to the idea that human mental faculties are general-purpose learning mechanisms.

Homeostasis and Negative Feedback
Homeostasis is one of the fundamental characteristics of living things. It refers to the maintenance of the internal environment within tolerable limits. All sorts of factors affect the suitability of our body fluids to sustain life; these include properties like temperature, salinity, acidity, and the concentrations of nutrients and wastes. Because these properties affect the chemical reactions that keep us alive, we have built-in physiological mechanisms to maintain them at desirable levels.

When a change occurs in the body, there are two general ways that the body can respond. In negative feedback, the body responds in such a way as to reverse the direction of change. Because this tends to keep things constant, it allows us to maintain homeostasis. On the other hand, positive feedback is also possible. This means that if a change occurs in some variable, the response is to change that variable even more in the same direction. This has a de-stabilizing effect, so it does not result in homeostasis. Positive feedback is used in certain situations where rapid change is desirable

To illustrate the components involved in negative feedback, we can use the example of a driver trying to stay near the speed limit. The desired value of a variable is called the set point. Here, the set point is a speed of 55 mph; in controlling body temperature, the set point would be 98.6 degrees. The control center is what monitors the variable and compares it with the set point. Here, the control center is the driver; for body temperature, it would be the hypothalamus of the brain. If the variable differs from the set point, the control center uses effectors to reverse the change. Here, the effector is the foot on the accelerator pedal; in controlling body temperature, it would include the glands that sweat and the muscles that shiver.

Functional Analysis – Team Approach

- Behavior as:
  - Communication
  - Serving a function

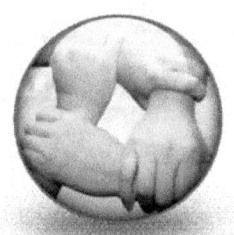

- Benefit of Team approacl
  - Different views of the beha
  - Wider range of ideas
  - Greater buy in

What is a "Functional Behavioral Assessment"?
Source: (Starin)

The term "Functional Behavioral Assessment" comes from what is called a "Functional Assessment" or "Functional Analysis" in the field of applied behavior analysis. This is the process of determining the cause (or "function") of behavior before developing an intervention. The intervention must be based on the hypothesized cause (function) of behavior.

Why do Functional Behavioral Assessments?
Failure to base the intervention on the specific cause (function) very often results in ineffective and unnecessarily restrictive procedures.

For example, consider the case of a young child who has learned that screaming is an effective way of avoiding or escaping unpleasant tasks. Using timeout in this situation would provide the child with exactly what he wants (avoiding the task) and is likely to make the problem worse, not better. Without an adequate functional behavioral assessment, we would not know the true function of the young child's screaming and therefore may select an inappropriate intervention.

How do you determine the cause or function of behavior?
There are three ways of getting at the function (cause) of the behavior:
- Interviews and rating scales.
- Direct and systematic observation of the person's behavior.
- Manipulating different environmental events to see how behavior changes.

The first two are generally referred to as functional assessments whereas the third is generally referred to as a functional analysis.

Several different interviews and rating scales have been developed to try to get at the function (cause) of behavior. However, reliability is usually poor and these should be used only as a starting point for systematic and direct observation of the person's behavior. Relying exclusively on interviews and rating scales should never be considered a functional assessment. Besides having poor reliability, it would never hold up in court with an expert witness.

A more reliable method involves directly observing the person's behavior in his or her natural environment and analyzing the behavior's antecedents (environmental events that immediately precede the problem behavior) and consequences (environmental events that immediately follow the problem behavior).

Types of Problem Behavior
Problem behavior typically falls into one or more of three general categories:
- Behavior that produces attention and other desired events (e.g., access to toys, desired activities).
- Behavior that allows the person to avoid or escape demands or other undesired events/activities.
- Behavior that occurs because of its sensory consequences (relieves pain, feels good, etc.).

The antecedents and consequences are analyzed to see which function(s) the behavior fulfills. Problem behavior can also serve more than one function, further complicating the matter. The interview, combined with direct observation of the behavior is what most people use in determining the function of the behavior. This is fine when the data collected on the antecedents and consequences is clear. Most of the time this is sufficient in determining the behavior's function(s).

Systematic Manipulation of Environment
In some cases, however, direct observation does not give a clear picture of the behavior's functions and systematically manipulating various environmental events becomes necessary. The most common way of systematically manipulating the environment is to put the person in several different situations and carefully observe how the behavior changes.

For example, to determine the function of screaming, we could arrange for attention to be given to the child each time she screams and measure how frequently screaming occurs. We could also make demands on the child, terminating them each time she screams and measure how frequently it occurs. In addition, we could leave the child alone and measure how often screaming occurs. If screaming is more frequent when attention is given, we hypothesize that it occurs to get attention. If screaming is more frequent when demands are made, we can assume that screaming has served to let the person escape or avoid demands. Finally, if screaming is more frequent when left alone, we can assume that it is occurring because of its sensory consequences. This third method should be reserved only for situations in which the functions of behavior are not clear through systematic and direct observation.

Intervention Plan

- Identify the function

- Identify alternative behaviors

- Teach/role model alternative behaviors

- Extinguish intervention when able

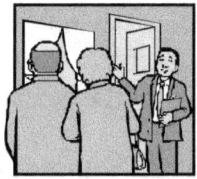

Source: (T. Mauro)
A Behavior Intervention Plan (BIP) takes the observations made in a Functional Behavioral Assessment and turns them into a concrete plan of action for managing behavior. A BIP may include ways to change the environment to keep behavior from starting in the first place, provide positive reinforcement to promote good behavior, employ planned ignoring to avoid reinforcing bad behavior, and provide supports needed so that the individual will not be driven to act out due to frustration or fatigue. When a behavior plan is

agreed to everyone commits to their role and consistent implementation. For this reason it is extremely important to closely monitor the interventions to insure no one is setting themselves or the plan up for failure by over committing.

A great intervention plan will address only one behavior at a time. Correctly identifying the function and providing alternative and more socially acceptable behavior is critical to its success.

All Behavior Intervention Plans should be seen as a work in progress. The team must be willing to acknowledge the whole or parts of the plan is not working and should be revised. The continuation of a bad plan can lead to much worst behaviors.

Ongoing Management Plan

- A biweekly review of plan

- Importance of tracking behavior (objectively)

Very few behavior intervention plans are perfect. Further as the client begins to respond to intervention the plan will need to be updated. Best practice, review plan at least every two weeks. This can be a formal or informal meeting usually conducted by the plan's coordinator. (A position established during the initial team meeting).

The fluidity of the plan and participants is key to its success. No one person, no matter how good the idea or intervention should dominate the planning process or the plan itself. Allow and encourage input from all members and recognize the plan as a group creation. In this way when your favorite part needs to be updated you will be less likely to take it personally.

Tacking behavior objectively is essential to recognizing the fruits of everyone's efforts. When teams use a methodical method of tracking the patients slight improvements are noted and celebrated. Very often when a plan is implement the expectation of complete and quick improvement lessens the recognition of the small improvements in the client's behavior. Remember, behavior modification is a slow process, by using objective and regular tracking these improvements are quickly noted.

If no improvement is seen with two or three days revisit the plan. If the behavior is severe the plan may need revisited even sooner.

Invite an outside expert in behavior modification if your team is unable to produce an improvement plan, previous plan for this client have failed, or you are not familiar with some of the details of the client's disorders.

Works Cited

About.com. (2008, May 02). *Alzheimer's Disease*. Retrieved Apr 2009, from http://alzheimers.about.com/od/diagnosisofalzheimers/a/crit eria.htm

Alz.org. (n.d.). *alz.org research center*. Retrieved Apr 2009, from http://www.alz.org/research/science/alzheimers_disease_ca uses.asp

Alzheimer's Association. (n.d.). *Meaningful Activities*. Retrieved Oct 2010, from http://www.alz.org/living_with_alzheimers_music_art_and _other_therapies.asp

Alzheimer's Association. (n.d.). *Stages of Alzheimer's*. Retrieved Apr 2010, from alz.org: http://www.alz.org/alzheimers_disease_stages_of_alzheime rs.asp

Alzheimer's Facts for Health. (n.d.). *What is the economic impact of Alzheimer's disease*. Retrieved Oct 2010, from alzheimers.factsforhealth.org: http://alzheimers.factsforhealth.org/what/impact.asp

Alzheimer's Review. (2009, Sept 24). *Alzheimer's disease: Causes, Symptoms, Treatment*. Retrieved Oct 2010, from http://alzheimers-review.blogspot.com/2009/09/progress-of-alzheimers-disease-timeline.html

American Music Therapy Association, Inc. (n.d.). *Music Therapy Fact Sheet*. Retrieved 2009 Apr, from http://www.musictherapy.org/factsheets/MT%20Alzheimer s%202006.pdf

Asociation for Humanistic Psychology. (n.d.). *Humanistic Psychology Overview*. Retrieved Oct 2010, from www.ahpweb.org: http://www.ahpweb.org/aboutahp/whatis.html

CBS Interactive Business Netword, Mark Warner. (2000, June). *DESIGNS for Validation Therapy*. Retrieved Oct 2010, from http://findarticles.com/p/articles/mi_m3830/is_6_49/ai_637 00200/

D. Rice, P. F. (1992). The Economic Burden of Alzheimer's Disease Care. *Data Watch #175*, 13.

Fisher Center for Alzheimer's Research Foundation. (2006, Nov 1). *Social Support*. Retrieved Apr 2009, from http://www.alzinfo.org/11/articles/caregiving-16

HelpGuide.org. (n.d.). *Managing Common Symptoms and Problems*. Retrieved Oct 2010, from Understand, Prevent and Resolve Challenges: http://helpguide.org/elder/alzheimers_behavior_problems.h tm

Itzhak, R. (1994, Aug). Retrieved Apr 2009, from Pub Med.gov: http://www.ncbi.nlm.nih.gov/pubmed/7888085

Mauro, T. (n.d.). *Special Needs Children*. Retrieved Oct 2010, from www.specialchildren.about.com: http://specialchildren.about.com/od/behavioranddiscipline/ g/BIP.htm

Mayo Clinic. (n.d.). *Alzheimer's disease*. Retrieved Apr 2010, from http://www.mayoclinic.com/health/alzheimers-stages/AZ00041

National Institute on Aging. (n.d.). *Alzheimer's Disease Genetics Fact Sheet*. Retrieved Oct 2010, from U.S. National Institutes of Health: http://www.nia.nih.gov/Alzheimers/Publications/geneticsfs. htm

National Institute on Aging. (n.d.). *Understanding Stages and Symptoms of Alzheimer's Disease*. Retrieved Oct 2010, from http://www.nia.nih.gov/Alzheimers/Publications/stages.htm

News, B. (2003, June 23). *BBC News*. Retrieved Apr 2009, from http://news.bbc.co.uk/2/hi/health/3014582.stm

O'Brien, J. (2007, Sept 19). *UCSF News Office*. Retrieved Apr 2009, from http://news.ucsf.edu/releases/early-alzheimers-disease-program-focuses-on-support-enrichment/

Science AAAS. (2006, May 2003). *Articles*. Retrieved Apr 2009, from
http://sageke.sciencemag.org/cgi/content/full/2006/8/pe10

Starin, S. (n.d.). *Functional Behavioral Assessments: What, Why, When, Where and Who?* Retrieved Oct 2010, from www.wrightslaw.com:
http://www.wrightslaw.com/info/discipl.fab.starin.htm

University of Pennsylvannia School of Medicine. (2007, March 20). *Alzheimer's Prevalence Tops Five Million in U.S.* Retrieved Apr 2009, from www.alz.org: http://www.alz.org

Wikipedia. (2010, May). *Classical Conditioning*. Retrieved May 2010, from The Free Encyclopedia:
http://en.wikipedia.org/wiki/Classical_conditioning

World Village. (2010, Oct). *The Pain and Pleasure Principal*. Retrieved Oct 2010, from http://worldvillage.com/the-pain-and-pleasure-principle

Chapter 5- Alzheimer's Disease: Evaluations & Treatments

Reason to Diagnose AD Early

- Safety
- Family stress and misunderstanding
- Early education of caregivers of how to handle patient
- Advance planning while patient is competent
- Client's and family's right to know

- Safety - driving, compliance, cooking, etc.
- Family stress and misunderstanding - blame, denial, etc.
- Early education of caregivers of how to handle client - choices, getting started.
- Advance planning while client is competent - will, proxy, power of attorney, advance directives.
- Client's and family's right to know.

Specific treatments now available, may delay nursing home placement longer if started earlier.

Source: (About.com Alzheimer's Disease)
Importance of Early Diagnosis for Alzheimer's Disease
- There are a number of important reasons to get a correct and early diagnosis for dementias such as Alzheimer's disease.

- Early diagnosis will identify the causes of the signs and symptoms a relative is displaying.
- Early diagnosis Alzheimer's allows prompt treatment of reversible symptoms. This can often lead to improvement of cognitive symptoms such as memory problems.
- Early diagnosis allows for the correct diagnosis of the dementia such as Alzheimer's.
- Early diagnosis of dementia allows for psychiatric symptoms to be identified and treated. Disease is not just about the illness itself. The psychological and social effects of Alzheimer's disease need to be addressed if there are signs and symptoms of such things as depression, agitation, or even psychosis. Early diagnosis and treatment can help prevent hospitalization and reduce impairment.
- Early diagnosis of dementias such as Alzheimer's gives people more time to make critical life decisions. These include financial planning.
- Putting into place legal frameworks to protect themselves and their family i.e. power of attorney, living wills and advanced medical directives.

Plans for Future Care

- Early diagnosis of dementia maximizes the safety of the person with Alzheimer's disease and their family. Diagnosis means that certain activities will need to be supervised, limited, or stopped. This includes driving9, the use of firearms for hunting and sport, and the use of heavy machinery, caring for the young or infirm. Some people will have to give up their work more quickly than others do, this will depend on the type of employment, their work roles, and the flexibility and support networks provided in their work place.
- Early diagnosis allows treatments for Alzheimer's disease that help slow its progression.
- Early diagnosis gives the person with Alzheimer's and their family more time to arm themselves with knowledge about this type of dementia and the best way to live with the disease. Knowledge really is power.

Do not avoid seeking medical input and assistance for Alzheimer's disease.

Early Recognition of AD: Consensus Statement (AAGP, AGS, Alzheimer's Association)

- AD continues to be missed as diagnosis

- AD is unrecognized and under-reported
  - patients do not realized
  - families tend to compensate

- Effective treatment and management techniques are available

Small et al., JAMA, 1997

Source: (Leutwyler, 2001)
Toward Early Diagnosis of Alzheimer's Disease
Certain brain structures may atrophy long before any symptoms of dementia surface, offering the chance to find and possibly treat the disease early.

All people forget some things sometimes. Everyone loses keys, miss appointments, and stash important papers in spots so secret they cannot, after the fact, remember where they are. It is entirely normal. But for many middle-aged and elderly individuals, such episodes prompt intense anxiety over Alzheimer's disease. The devastating neurodegenerative disease slowly corrodes the brain until memories, moods, and many other cognitive traits are permanently lost. And perhaps most frightening, it seems to creep up on its victims without much warning.

Researchers have over the years devised psychological screening tests to try to identify people in the early stages of Alzheimer's disease. Apart from memory loss, there are nine other warning signs among them difficulty performing familiar tasks; problems with language, such as remembering words; disorientation in time and space; and changes in personality. Scientists have also noted that susceptible people appear to have a greater sensitivity to the drug tropicamide, which is ordinarily used to dilate the pupils in a routine eye exam. But for the most part, diagnosis has been a process of elimination.

Recently, however, a team of scientists from University College London and the Imperial College School of Medicine described in the journal *The Lancet* a new way to actually predict who will develop Alzheimer's as early as three years before symptoms appear. Nick Fox, Martin Rossor and their colleagues discovered distinctive patterns of progressive atrophy in the brains of pre-diagnosis Alzheimer's patients by taking series of MRI images. "It raises the hope that we might one day be able to intervene with therapy at a very early stage," the authors write, "before the devastating cognitive decline of the disease has already become established."

In fact, several early or preventive therapies have shown promise in animal studies. Researchers have devised vaccines that appear to prevent the formation of amyloid plaques associated with the disease. And scientists have removed existing plaques in mice by applying anti-plaque antibodies directly to the animals' brains. Using gene therapy, other experimentalists have successfully restored axons the vital fibers that relay messages between brain cells in aged monkeys. Stalling or stopping the progress of Alzheimer's disease might become possible several decades out.

So to try to pinpoint the very earliest structural brain damage associated with Alzheimer's, Fox and colleagues chose to study the offspring of patients with the familial form of the disease. These people have a 50 percent chance of developing Alzheimer's at a fairly young age. They recruited four such symptom-free individuals, as well as 20 people having a probable diagnosis of familial or sporadic Alzheimer's disease and 20 of their spouses as controls.

All underwent annual serial MRI brain scans in addition to comprehensive physical examinations over the course of five to eight years. The scientists very carefully matched the MRIs from individuals so that they could map volume changes over time, creating what are known as voxel compression maps. "Voxel compression mapping provides a valuable technique for in-vivo monitoring of the progression of Alzheimer's disease," Fox says.

As it turned out, the four at-risk subjects all progressed to Alzheimer's over the course of the study, providing the scientists with a clear view of the disease in its very beginnings. All of the subjects lost cerebral volume, but the rate of that loss was much greater in the people with mild to moderate Alzheimer's. In this respect, the four at-risk individuals more closely resembled the Alzheimer's patients at the study's start: their initial median rate of atrophy was significantly higher than that of the controls, well before they showed symptoms.

In addition to the different rates of loss, the scientists discovered that the various subject groups also exhibited different patterns of loss. In the Alzheimer's patients, widespread regions of gray and white matter were consistently wasted; only the primary motor and sensory cortices, brain stem, and cerebellum were spared. The changes in the healthy controls were also somewhat diffuse. But in the four at-risk subjects, progressive atrophy was most pronounced in the posterior cingulate, the parietal lobe and, in particular, the medial temporal lobe.

The scientists warn that "some caution is needed in extrapolating results found in familial Alzheimer's disease to the more common sporadic Alzheimer's disease." Nevertheless, their findings accord well with other lines of study into the disease's histological changes (plaques, tangles, etc.), which probably precede any structural changes. "We have been able to show a presymptomatic phase of three years or more of increased rates of tissue loss," the authors explain. "The recognition of a presymptomatic phase, which extends beyond the medial temporal lobe, implies that structural changes might start earlier and are more widely distributed that previously appreciated."

Need for Better Screening and Early Assessment Tools

- Genetic vulnerability testing

- Early recognition
  - List of 10
  - Key points for Health Care Providers

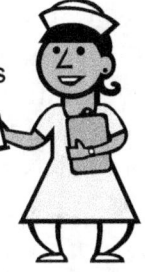

Source: (Alzheimer's Association)

The Alzheimer's Association has developed a list of warning signs that include common symptoms of Alzheimer's disease.

Individuals who exhibit several of these symptoms should see a physician for a complete examination:

- Memory loss that affects job skills.
- Difficulty performing familiar tasks.
- Problems with language.
- Disorientation to time and place (getting lost).
- Poor or decreased judgment.
- Problems with abstract thinking.
- Misplacing things.
- Changes in mood or behavior.
- Changes in personality.
- Loss of initiative.

Key Points about Alzheimer's Disease

For Health Care Providers

- Although changes in memory or cognition may accompany normal aging, significant impairment and disability are not a part of normal aging.

- It is important for clinicians, as well as patients and family members, to recognize symptoms that should trigger an initial assessment for dementia.
- Some causes of dementia can be treated effectively to eliminate or greatly improve cognitive performance.
- Among older persons, depression and interactions from multiple medications are two common and highly treatable causes of dementia symptoms.
- The prolonged course of deterioration found in many dementias takes a major emotional, psychiatric, and physical toll among family members and caregivers.

An initial assessment for dementia can

- Lead to effective treatment of causes.
- Prevent unnecessary and possibly harmful treatment resulting from misdiagnosis.
- Avoid the trauma of a diagnosis of dementia or Alzheimer's disease where it does not exist.

For Patients
- Dementia is different from normal aging. Only certain tests can show that difference. Symptoms that suggest Alzheimer's disease or a related dementia should be brought to the attention of the family's health care provider as soon as possible.
- Some memory and other problems can improve or disappear with appropriate treatment.
- Although there is not yet a clearly effective treatment for Alzheimer's disease, resources are available to help patients and families cope with this condition and prepare for the future.
- Order the consumer booklet, *Early Alzheimer's Disease: Client and Family Guide* from the U.S. Government's Agency for Health Care Policy and Research. It provides information about the early stages of Alzheimer's disease and similar illnesses. It also includes a list of resources where readers can find out more about the medical, financial, and social support services that are available in their communities.

Symptoms that may Indicate Dementia
- Does the person have increased difficulty with any of the activities listed below? Positive findings in any of these areas generally indicate the need for further assessment for the presence of dementia.
- Learning and retaining new information. *For example:* is more repetitive; has more trouble remembering recent conversations, events, appointments; more frequently misplaces objects.
- Handling complex tasks. *For example:* has more trouble following a complex train of thought, performing tasks that require many steps such as balancing a checkbook or cooking a meal.
- Reasoning ability. *For example:* is unable to respond with a reasonable plan to problems at work or home, such as knowing what to do if the bathroom flooded; shows uncharacteristic disregard for rules of social conduct.
- Spatial ability and orientation. *For example:* has trouble driving, organizing objects around the house, and finding his or her way around familiar places.
- Language. *For example:* has increasing difficulty with finding the words to express what he or she wants to say and with following conversations.
- Behavior. *For example:* appears more passive and less responsive; is more irritable than usual; is more suspicious than usual; misinterprets visual or auditory stimuli. In addition to failure to arrive at the right time for appointments; the clinician can look for difficulty discussing current events in an area on interest and changes in behavior and dress. It might also be helpful to follow up on areas of concern by asking the client or family members relevant questions.

Alzheimer's Top Ten Warning Signs
(Alzheimer Association)

1. Recent memory loss affecting job
2. Difficulty performing familiar tasks
3. Problems with language
4. Disorientation to time or place
5. Poor or decreased judgment
6. Problems with abstract thinking
7. Misplacing things
8. Changes in mood or behavior
9. Changes in personality
10. Loss of initiative

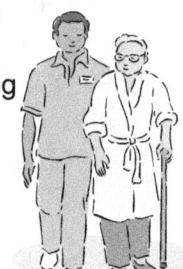

Need for Brief Screening Test for Alzheimer's Disease

• Recent evidence of benefits of anti-cholinesterase agents in treatment of mild Alzheimer's Disease
   – Improvement of cognition
   – Slowing of progression

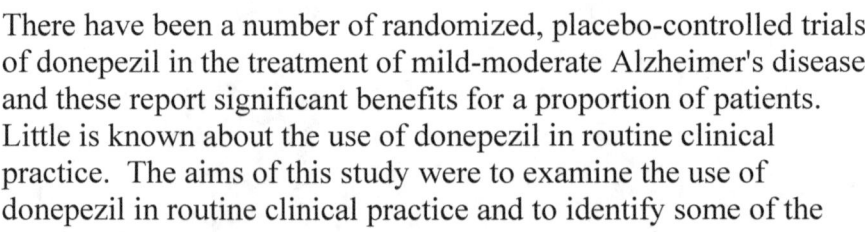

There have been a number of randomized, placebo-controlled trials of donepezil in the treatment of mild-moderate Alzheimer's disease and these report significant benefits for a proportion of patients. Little is known about the use of donepezil in routine clinical practice. The aims of this study were to examine the use of donepezil in routine clinical practice and to identify some of the practical and resource implications associated with treatment. A number of areas were examined against published guidelines including assessment, diagnosis, and initiation of treatment, monitoring, and discontinuation of treatment. This was a retrospective case note study involving patients with mild-moderate Alzheimer's disease over a one-year period. One hundred and seventeen patients were commenced on donepezil and 93 successfully completed three months of treatment. Of these, 47% demonstrated an improvement in cognition, activities of daily living or career observation, (or a combination).

In addition to drug/medications one can also start the client on increased daily exercise, change eating pattern, and encourage cognitively developmental activities (i.e., reading, puzzles, etc.)

Available Screening Tests

- MMSE   10 -- 15 min
  - Too long
- 7-Minute Screen   7 – 10 min
  - Too complex
- Clock Drawing Test   2 – 4 min
  - Not sensitive
- Mini-cognitive   3 – 5 min
  - Complex scoring, unclear adequacy
- Memory Impairment Screen   4 min
  - Need for slightly shorter, easier test

- A suitably accurate test taking less than 2 minutes not available

These assessments were reviewed in chapter 3. Refer to that chapter for details on each of these assessments if needed.

Bottom Line: the need for a quick, sensitive, and reliable assessment. One should also emphasize the need for good record keeping as a general decline in functioning may provide medical personnel with indication of Alzheimer's onset.

Brief Alzheimer's Screening

- Repeat these three words: "apple, table, penny".
- So you will remember these words, repeat them again, twice.
- What is today's date?
  - 1 point if within 2 days.
- "Name as many animals as you can in 30 seconds, GO!"
  - 1 point for naming 10 animals
- "What were the 3 words I asked you to repeat?" (no prompts)
  - 1 for each word,
- TOTAL (max = 5)
  - A score of 4 or 5 indicate a very low likelihood of dementia.
  - A score of 2 or 3 suggests that more testing is needed.
  - A score of 0 or 1 indicate a very high likelihood of dementia.
  - (palm-pilot scoring under development)

- If score of 2 or 3:
  - Spell World Backwards
  - Draw a Clock (gives some impression of visuospatial problems)
- If continued difficulties, ask questions about ADLs

This is just one possible screening. Note that with practice the client will improve in these areas. Giving this assessment too often may lead to a practice effect.

Physical/Neurological Examination

- Blood Pressure
- Systemic Disorders
- Cranial Nerves
  - Olfactory dysfunction, poor eye tracking
  - hearing, vision deficits
- Sensory Deficits
  - Proprioception, vibration
- Deep Tendon Reflexes
  - Brisk, check for focal reflexes

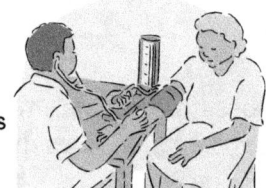

Source: (Wrongdiagnosis.com)

Systemic Disorders: Any condition that occurs in a system of the body.

Types of Systemic Disorders: Mitochondrial disorders, Metabolic disorders, Aging, Diabetes, Insulin Resistance, Metabolic Syndrome, Systemic lupus erythematous, Diabetes Insipidus, Cushing's syndrome, Hypertension, Hypercholesterolemia, Hemochromatosis, Wilson's Disease, Addisonian crisis, Alkalosis, Acidosis, Anaphylaxis, Hangover, and Pituitary conditions.

Olfactory Dysfunction: A dysfunction that occurs to the sense of smell.

Some causes:

- Allergic rhinitis.
- Viral rhinitis.
- Idiopathic.
- Anatomic blockage of nares.
- Head trauma.
- Alzheimer's disease.
- Parkinson's disease.
- Head trauma.

Proprioception — from Latin *proprius*, meaning "one's own," and *perception* — is one of the human senses. There are between nine and 21 in all, depending on which sense researcher you ask. Rather than sensing external reality, proprioception is the sense of the orientation of one's limbs in space. This is distinct from the sense of balance, which derives from the fluids in the inner ear, and is called *equilibrioception*. Proprioception is what police officers test when they pull someone over and suspect drunkenness. Without proprioception, we would need to consciously watch our feet to make sure that we stay upright while walking.

Proprioception does not come from any specific organ, but from the nervous system as a whole. Its input comes from sensory receptors distinct from tactile receptors — nerves from inside the body rather than on the surface. Proprioceptive ability can be trained, as can any motor activity.

Without proprioception, drivers would be unable to keep their eyes on the road while driving, as they would need to pay attention to the position of their arms and legs while working the pedals and steering wheel. And I would not be able to type this article without staring at the keys. If you happen to be snacking while reading this article, you would be unable to put food into your mouth without taking breaks to judge the position and orientation of your hands.

Learning any new motor skill involves training our proprioceptive sense. Anything that involves moving our arms or legs in a precise way without looking at them invokes it — baseball, basketball, painting, you name it. Proprioception is often overlooked as one of the senses because it is so automatic that our conscious mind barely notices it. It is one of the oldest senses, probably even more evolutionarily ancient than smell.

Among other reasons, proprioception is known to be a distinct sense because there are cases in which the proprioceptive ability is absent in a client. This means that proprioception uses dedicated brain ware. Proprioception-disabled patients can only walk by paying attention to where they put their legs. Thankfully, this condition is extremely rare.

Deep Tendon Reflex (DTR), a brisk contraction of a muscle in response to a sudden stretch induced by a sharp tap by a finger or rubber hammer on the tendon of insertion of the muscle. Absence of the reflex may be caused by damage to the muscle, peripheral nerve, nerve roots, or spinal cord at that level. A hyperactive reflex may indicate disease of the pyramidal tract above the level of the reflex arc being tested. Generalized hyperactivity of DTRs may be caused by hyperthyroidism. Kinds of DTRs include Achilles tendon reflex, biceps reflex, brachioradialis reflex, patellar reflex, and triceps reflex. Also called myostatic reflex, tendon reflex.

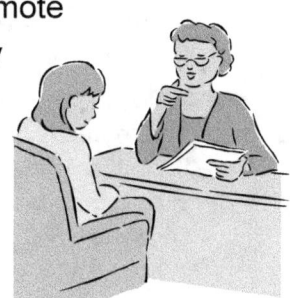

Neuropsychological Testing
(WAIS, Wechsler)

- Memory: Short-term, Remote
- Verbal Function, Fluency
- Visuo-spatial Function
- Attention
- Executive Function
- Abstract Thinking
- Account For Education

Definition
The Wechsler adult intelligence scale (WAIS) is an individually administered measure of intelligence, intended for adults aged 16–89.

Source: (Encyclopedia of Mental Disorders)
Purpose
The WAIS is intended to measure human intelligence reflected in both verbal and performance abilities. Dr. David Wechsler, a clinical psychologist, believed that intelligence is a global construct, reflecting a variety of measurable skills and should be considered in the context of the overall personality. The WAIS is also administered as part of a test battery to make inferences about personality and pathology, both through the content of specific answers and patterns of subtest scores.

Besides being utilized as an intelligence assessment, the WAIS is used in neuropsychological evaluation, specifically with regard to brain dysfunction. Large differences in verbal and nonverbal intelligence may indicate specific types of brain damage.

The WAIS is also administered for diagnostic purposes. Intelligence quotient (IQ) scores reported by the WAIS can be used as part of the diagnostic criteria for mental retardation, specific learning disabilities, and attention-deficit/hyperactivity disorder (ADHD).

Laboratory Tests (routine)

- Blood Tests
  - electrolytes, liver, kidney function tests, glucose
  - thyroid function tests
  - vitamin B12, folate
  - complete blood count, ESR
  - VDRL, HIV
  - EKG
- Chest x-ray
- Urinalysis
- MRI

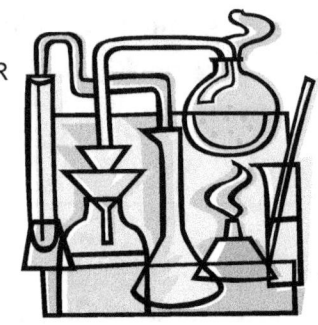

These slides are provided for general information to alert the health care provider to the numerous and proper diagnosing procedures. This information may be a good starting point to advocate for a client.

Special Laboratory Tests

- Functional Brain Imaging
- EEG
- Reaction Times (slowed in the elderly, especially when complex response is required)
- Heavy Metal Screen
- Genotyping
  - Early onset
  - Family history

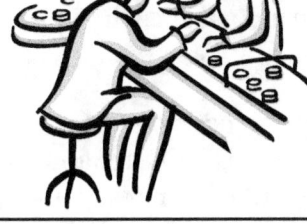

Genetic Testing to Predict AD?

- Family members want it
  - They consider recommendations against genetic testing to be "paternalistic"
- Family members may make more powerful financial decisions based on this knowledge than relevance of insurance companies implementing changes in actuarial calculations
- Those at risk can seek more frequent testing
  - This is the best opportunity for early recognition
- Those at risk will be better advocates for research
- Specific preventive treatments can be developed for each genetic factor

Source: (National Institute on Aging)
Alzheimer's disease is a common cause of age-related dementia, but not all dementia is due to Alzheimer's. Among all cases of

Alzheimer's, only a minority are the inherited form, which can either be early-onset (symptoms before age 65) or late-onset.

Genetic testing is available for early-onset Alzheimer's, but only about 2% of familial Alzheimer's is the early-onset type. Early-onset of familial Alzheimer's has a dominant inheritance pattern. This means that a person only needs to inherit one copy of the changed gene to get the disease. If one of your parents had a change in one of these genes, you have a 50% chance of having the same change, and each of your children has a 50% chance of inheriting it from you.

Using the genetic test to predict if a healthy person will get Alzheimer's is NOT reliable. Some people with "high-risk" results do not get Alzheimer's, while others get Alzheimer's even though they do not have "high-risk" results.

Imagine receiving a test result saying you will get Alzheimer's and then you worry and worry but never get the disease! For this reason, genetic testing to predict if you will develop late-onset Alzheimer's is not advisable. You should talk to your doctor about what makes sense based on your family history.

Genetic testing is performed to see if a person has certain genes that show whether he or she is more likely to be at risk for certain diseases or conditions. Not everyone who has a risk for a disease develops that disease. Genetic tests can be performed on a sample of blood, hair, skin or other tissue. Commonly, a procedure called a buccal smear uses a small brush or cotton swab to collect a sample of cells from the inside surface of the cheek. The sample is sent to a laboratory for analysis.

Alzheimer's disease is a type of dementia that develops over a period of years and leads to a progressive decline in mental function. Alzheimer's disease is considered familial or nonfamilial. Nonfamilial Alzheimer's disease accounts for about 75 percent of the cases and does not appear to run in families. Familial Alzheimer's disease is less common and is found in multiple members of a family. Four major types of familial

Alzheimer's disease have been identified. Types 1, 3, and 4 are classified as early-onset Alzheimer's disease because their signs and symptoms appear before age 65. Type 2 is classified as late-onset Alzheimer's disease because its signs and symptoms appear after age 65.

Researchers have identified three genes that cause early-onset forms of Alzheimer's disease. The genes that cause late-onset familial Alzheimer's disease are not as clear.

Things to Consider
- A genetic defect cannot be repaired, generally cannot be treated, and may cause anxiety and questions with no clear answers.
- Genetic testing for a high risk of late onset Alzheimer's disease cannot accurately predict who will develop the disease.
- Testing positive by genetic testing for Alzheimer's disease does not mean you will definitely develop the disease.
- Testing negative by genetic testing for Alzheimer's disease does not guarantee that you will not develop the disease.
- Testing positive by genetic testing for Alzheimer's disease may lead to discrimination affecting your ability to plan for your advancing age.

Results
Will I live longer if I have this procedure?
No, there is no scientific evidence genetic testing for Alzheimer's disease will prolong life.

Will genetic testing for Alzheimer's disease improve my quality of life?
No, there is no scientific evidence that genetic testing for Alzheimer's disease will improve quality of life. It may cause anxiety and testing positive does not mean you will develop the disease. However, it may allow you to make plans for your advancing age.

Will genetic testing for Alzheimer's disease make my symptoms better?
No, there is no scientific evidence that genetic testing for Alzheimer's disease will make my symptoms better.

How safe is this for me?
There is very little risk from having a blood sample taken from a vein. You may develop a bruise at the puncture site. In rare cases, the vein may become inflamed. If you have a bleeding problem or take blood-thinning medication, you should tell your health care provider before the blood sample is drawn.

Many of the risks associated with genetic testing involve the emotional, social, or financial consequences of the test results.

Minor reported complications:
- Bruising after having a blood sample drawn
- There have been no reported complications related to the swab from inside the cheek

Major reported complications:
None reported

Comparison
Currently, there is no alternative testing to predict whether some one will develop Alzheimer's disease.

Cost
The cost can vary depending on the laboratory doing the test and the area of the country where you have the test done. The cost may or may not be covered by your health benefits plan.

Treatment - Behavioral

- Should be tried first, before medications

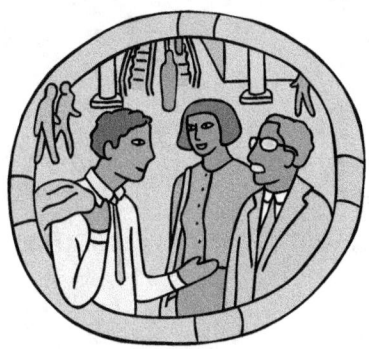

As a psychologist, I should also throw a plug in for behavioral approaches to the demented client. Treatment guidelines generally recommend using behavioral approaches first, before medications are used. These techniques may seem obvious, but you should ask family members what they have been trying already---families have varying degrees of sophistication in this matter.

The most important thing you can tell families is that they should NOT argue with the demented individual. This typically only leads to tears or to an escalation of the behavior. Perhaps the simplest thing to do is simply to provide the demented client with an environment that is more accommodating of their behaviors.

Treatment - Pharmacologic

- Behavioral problems are most important
- Secondary to...
  - Agitation
  - Depression
  - Delusions
  - Aggression
- Improvements are usually modest

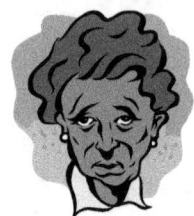

Once you have some idea of the type of dementia you are working with, you can consider a treatment. Very often the behavioral problems of dementia warrant primary attention and may be secondary to agitation, depression, delusions, or aggression. All of these can show some improvement with treatment. But improvements tend to be modest.

Although there is currently no way to cure Alzheimer's disease or stop its progression, researchers are making encouraging advances in Alzheimer's treatment, including medications and non-drug approaches to improve symptom management. When physicians develop treatment plans, they often consider cognitive and behavioral symptoms separately.

Source: (Alzheimer's Disease: Causes, Symptoms, Treatment, 2010)

Cognitive Symptoms

Cognitive symptoms include problems with thought processes like memory, language, and judgment. Two kinds of medications have been approved by the U.S. Food and Drug Administration for treatment of cognitive symptoms of Alzheimer's disease:

Cholinesterase inhibitors increase the levels of acetylcholine in the brain, which plays a key role in memory and learning. This kind of drug postpones the worsening of symptoms for 6 to 12 months in about half of the people who take it. Cholinesterase inhibitors most commonly prescribed for mild to moderate Alzheimer's disease include Aricept (donezepil HCL), Exelon (rivastigmine), and Razadyne (galantamine). Because of varying side effects and possible interactions with other medications, doctors may try different cholinesterase inhibitors until the most effective one is found for the individual.

Namenda (memantine) regulates glutamate in the brain, which plays a key role in processing information. This drug is used to treat moderate to severe Alzheimer's disease and may delay the worsening of symptoms in some people.

Cholinesterase inhibitors can be started as soon as Alzheimer's symptoms appear -- in fact, they are most effective in the early stages of the disease. When a physician determines that the cholinesterase inhibitor is no longer effective, he or she often recommends tapering off the cholinesterase inhibitor and introducing memantine. Sometimes, memantine and a cholinesterase inhibitor are taken simultaneously during the moderate stage of the disease.

Behavioral Symptoms
Often the most challenging for caregivers, behavioral symptoms include agitation, suspicion, and depression. Although caregivers often take personally the behaviors exhibited toward them, it is important to remember that behavioral symptoms are just as much a result of damage to brain cells as are cognitive symptoms.

Some medications are useful for managing behavioral symptoms. For instance, anti-anxiety medications can treat agitation and aggression, while anti-psychotic medications have been used to address suspicion and paranoia. However, the risk of drug reactions and/or interactions runs high among those with Alzheimer's, so caution should be used when medications are prescribed to deal with behavioral issues. A combination of drug and non-drug treatments often works best.

Non-drug treatments involve analyzing the behavior, identifying what may have triggered it, and devising an approach that changes either the person's environment or the caregiver's reaction to the behavior.

For example, excessive noise can worsen agitation in individuals with Alzheimer's. Simply creating a calmer environment may eliminate the behavior. Likewise, when caregivers become angry in response to a difficult behavior, this usually only upsets the person with Alzheimer's and increases the behavior's frequency. Reacting in a calm, controlled manner can reduce the tension long enough to distract the person to a more pleasant activity, such as looking at a family photo album or listening to a favorite kind of music.

While physicians are skilled at prescribing medications to treat behavioral symptoms, they may not be familiar with non-drug interventions. Most caregivers learn about behavior management through their own research and by connecting with other caregivers through support groups and online support networks.

Treatment - Pharmacologic

- Antidepressants
- Anticonvulsants
- Benzodiazepines
- Psychostimulants
- Cognitive Enhancers

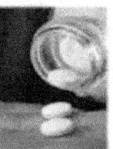
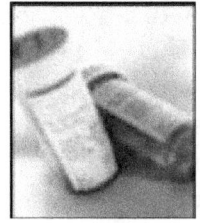

Source: (Felthous, 2007)

Virtually every class of psychotropic medication has been used in the treatment of these behaviors. These include antidepressants, neuroleptics, anticonvulsants, benzodiazepines, stimulants, and now the cognitive enhancers donepezil (Aricept), rivastigmine (exelon), and galantamine (reminyl).

Deciding whether and when to treat Alzheimer's disease with medications can be a difficult decision. Assessing the severity of your condition can help you decide whether medications are right for you. Consider the following when making your decision:

- Symptoms interfere with daily living and are more bothersome than the potential side effects of the medication, so taking medications may be a good choice.
- Disruptive behaviors may be manageable without medications. If behavior problems can be managed in other ways, may be able to avoid treatment with medication and the side effects and costs that come with it.
- Treatment with a cholinesterase inhibitor may reduce the burden on caregivers by producing small improvements in memory and general ability to function. For example, one may be able to remember friends' names better and be able to dress ones self with less difficulty.
- Medications for Alzheimer's disease do not work for everyone who takes them, and their effectiveness is not always dramatic. Even if they do initially reduce symptoms, the medications eventually will no longer control the progressive symptoms of memory problems, behavioral and personality changes, and thinking problems caused by Alzheimer's disease.
- Medications can relieve symptoms and restore ability to function. They may temporarily improve physical and mental health by taking medications. While medications may reduce the severity of Alzheimer's symptoms— thinking and memory problems, and personality changes— they will not completely eliminate the symptoms nor will they prevent the disease from progressing.

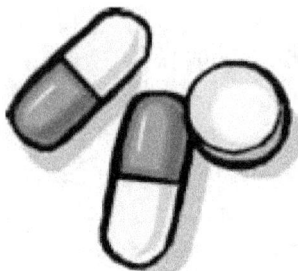

Source: (Curtis, 2007)

With all these medications to choose from, it becomes important to develop a strategy in approaching these behaviorally and medically complicated patients.

Generally, it is best to select one problematic behavior that to be controlled above all others.

To do this, ask:

- Is it behavior driven by paranoia and psychosis to be treated?
- If it seems to be depression or severe apathy, then the medication tried may be an antidepressant or a psychostimulant.
- If it is emotional liability or disinhibition in the absence of psychosis, then an anticonvulsant or mood stabilizer may be the best choice.
- If agitation without psychosis is the main concern than any of the above may be a reasonable choice.

A class of drugs widely prescribed for people suffering from dementia is leading to the premature deaths of thousands of patients every year, according to research published today.

Campaigners branded the continued use of the sedatives, called neuroleptics, a national scandal after a five-year study revealed that people with Alzheimer's disease and other forms of dementia are twice as likely to die if they are prescribed them.

Neuroleptics are widely prescribed to help control symptoms of Alzheimer's and dementia including agitation, hallucinations and erratic behavior, despite only being licensed for use in people suffering from schizophrenia. The research suggests they are of little benefit to patients with milder symptoms, greatly increase their risk of dying prematurely, and that 45% of Alzheimer's patients in care homes are prescribed a neuroleptic drug.

A group of 165 Alzheimer's patients were randomly assigned to take one of three types of neuroleptic drugs, or a placebo. After two years 45% of those who took the real drugs had died compared with 22% who were given the placebo.

The King's College London researchers who undertook the project, funded by the Alzheimer's Research Trust, found that after three years 65% of those on the drugs had died compared with 38% of those on placebos. After 42 months 75% of those on the drugs had died compared with 60% on the placebo. On average patients who were on the drugs died six months earlier.

Clive Ballard, professor of age-related disorders at King's and the lead researcher, said that not only were people more likely to die but they also suffered severe side-effects including stroke, chest infections and falls.

"If this was a massive increase in mortality in children there would be an outcry. Older people are not seen as a priority. These sedatives are being used because the services cannot cope with people who are in a distressed state. There are ways to avoid them but it would involve training of staff, which is costly."

In 2004 the medicines watchdog issued a warning that two types of neuroleptics, olanzapine and risperidone, should not be given to

Alzheimer's patients because of an increased risk of stroke and death.

Despite this, in 2005 the Alzheimer's Society presented evidence that 100,000 people suffering from dementia were being prescribed a neuroleptic drug.

Neil Hunt, chief executive of the society, said: "Neuroleptics have been used as a dangerous fix for 'challenging behavior' in people with dementia for too long. They are not licensed for use among people with dementia, but continue to be hugely over-prescribed. It is a national scandal that people are being sedated in this way ... These drugs must be a last resort, only used when all other methods have failed to alleviate the most distressing symptoms of dementia."

Rebecca Wood, chief executive of the Alzheimer's Research Trust, said: "These results are deeply troubling and highlight the urgent need to develop better treatments."

The Medicines and Healthcare products Regulatory Agency (MHRA), which is responsible for the safety of medications, said neuroleptics, were not licensed for use to treat dementia. "The MHRA continues to monitor the unlicensed use of neuroleptics in the treatment of patients with Alzheimer's disease and will carefully review this new study to see what further action may be necessary."

Professor Mayur Lakhani, chairman of the Royal College of General Practitioners, said: "We would like to reassure patients, relatives, and careers that neuroleptic drugs are not routinely prescribed to patients with dementia, and are used only as a last resort when patients suffer from severe episodes."

Antidepressants in Dementia

- Trazodone for agitation and aggression, but not for depression
- SSRI's make theoretical sense because of serotonin deficiency
- Tricyclics not for "agitation"

Source: (Martinon-Torres)
Insufficient evidence from randomized, placebo-controlled studies to support a recommendation that trazodone should be prescribed, or not prescribed, for BPSD.

The rationale for using trazodone is that it is a sedating atypical serotonergic antidepressant with a low rate of adverse effects and some behavioral and psychological symptoms in people with dementia (BPSD) are associated with serotonergic dysfunction. The conclusion is based on limited data from two small studies. The larger of the studies, conducted in 73 patients with Alzheimer's disease, showed no beneficial effect of trazodone at all. A smaller cross-over study in patients with frontal lobe dementia showed a trend for reduction in some symptoms in the first study period. Larger, longer studies are needed to explore the efficacy, effectiveness, and safety of trazodone.

Trazodone might worsen the confusion of an elderly client with Alzheimer's.
Depression is common in people with Alzheimer's disease and doctors will often use antidepressant medication to treat it.

SSRI Antidepressant Medications
Depression with or without agitation can be treated with medications such as those in the SSRI group of medications. SSRI stands for Selective Serotonin Reuptake Inhibitors. This describes the way in which the drug works in the brain. SSRI medications have been found to be effective in the treatment of depression for people with Alzheimer's disease. These medications include: Prozac, Zoloft, Lexapro, Paxil, and Celexa.

Side effects of SRRI medications include can sweating, tremors, nervousness, insomnia or somnolence, dizziness, and various gastrointestinal and sexual disturbances.

Depression with Agitation and Alzheimer's disease
Trazodone (Desyrel) can be very good for depression with agitation because of its sedating qualities. Initial dosage 25 to 50 mg daily. Increased to 100 to 300 mg daily in two or three doses. Side effects include over sedation, less commonly dizziness, orthostasis, headache, cardiac irritability. Very rarely priapism.

Tricyclic Antidepressants for Alzheimer's
Another group of antidepressants used in the treatment of depression in Alzheimer's disease are called tricyclic antidepressants. Examples of this drug group are desipramine (Norpramin) and nortriptyline (Pamelor).

Desipramine (Norpramin) is good for people with Alzheimer's disease and depression who have more apathetic features as the drug tends to be activating. Dosage initial is from 10 to 25 mg in the morning.to a maximum 150 mg in the morning.

Side Effects of Desipramine include Tachycardia.
Nortriptyline (Pamelor) tends to have a more sedative effects so may be useful for people with Alzheimer's disease who are depressed but agitated and who may also suffer from sleep disturbances such as insomnia.

Dosage may initially be 10 mg at bedtime. If well tolerated dose can be increased to 10 to 40 mg per day given in two doses.

New research suggests that an antidepressant (citalopram) may perform as well as a commonly-prescribed antipsychotic (risperidone) in the alleviation of severe agitation and psychotic symptoms of dementia.

Moreover, the antidepressant was associated with significantly lower adverse side effects.

The finding surprised researchers and may represent a new direction in drug treatment for psychotic disorders related to dementia in the elderly.

However, additional studies are needed to replicate the findings. In the meantime, second generation antipsychotics continue to be a first-line pharmacological treatment, despite growing scientific evidence that they can be associated with serious side effects, including death.

The study, published in the online American Journal of Geriatric Psychiatry (in advance of the November 2007 issue), is believed to be the first head-to-head comparison of an SSRI (selective serotonin reuptake inhibitor) with one of the more commonly prescribed second generation antipsychotics in older, non-depressed patients.

"We are encouraged by this early data, but we need to learn more in further trials that include a placebo group before we can say with confidence that antidepressants are an effective and safe treatment for agitation and psychosis in patients suffering from dementia," says lead investigator Dr. Bruce Pollock, who teamed up with colleague Dr. Benoit Mulsant to conduct the study.

Drs. Pollock and Mulsant conducted a double-blind randomized control trial of citalopram (antidepressant) and risperidone (antipsychotic) to compare the efficacy and safety of the two drugs in 103 patients who were hospitalized with psychiatric disturbances related to dementia at the University of Pittsburgh Medical Center.

The researchers were surprised to find that citalopram and risperidone had similar efficacy in reducing psychosis (hallucinations, delusions, suspicious thoughts) and agitation.

Overall, there was a 32 percent reduction of symptoms with citalopram and a 35 percent reduction with risperidone. Citalopram was associated with a significantly lower burden of adverse side effects, such as sedation, tension, and apathy. Total side effect burden scores increased 19 percent for risperidone and decreased by 4 percent with citalopram.

"We did not expect that an antidepressant would have so-called antipsychotic properties," adds Dr. Mulsant. It reinforces the belief that psychosis and agitation have a different neurochemistry in older patients with dementia and in younger patients with schizophrenia, even though both groups of patients are currently treated with the same medications (antipsychotics).

Cognitive Enhancers
Acetylcholine Esterase Inhibitor (AchEI)

- FDA approved for Alzheimer's
  - Side effects: GI upset, nausea, diarrhea, sleep
  - Consider for Lewy Body
  - Expensive!
  - How will you know they've been helpful?
    - Another argument for cognitive screening test
    - Document baseline level of functioning

Finally, no talk about the pharmacological treatment of dementia would be complete nowadays without some mention of the cognitive enhancers.

So far, there are three of them. They have been approved for mild to moderate Alzheimer's disease. These medications seem to delay the progression of Alzheimer's disease although they do not reverse it. There have been some studies to suggest that they can delay nursing home placement by 12 months or more.

There are no randomized controlled studies using the cognitive enhancers with the other types of dementias but these studies are underway. There are also studies regarding their use in patients with more advanced cases of Alzheimer's but data are pending.

At any rate, one should familiarize one's self with their most common side effects before using them. They ALL can cause GI upset, nausea, loose stools, and disturb sleep or even cause nightmares. This effect seems to be dose related.

These medications have become more popular in patients with Lewy Body Dementia, and they have been reported to help with the psychosis associated with that disorder. They are expensive! The question one will always have after therapy has been on them is did they help or not? (Another argument for using a cognitive screening test...)

Hope is on the horizon, however, in the form of recent advances such as the completion of the Human Genome Project, modern molecular biology, and new brain-imaging technologies. Researchers have an unprecedented view into the workings of the brain, which has in turn helped define the chemistry of the brain and suggested gene targets for the discovery of cognitive enhancers, drugs that sharpen mental faculties.

Source: (Halim)
CREB: The Memory Switch?
The brain is a complex network of neurons that communicate with each other through chemical signals. This process can trigger the synthesis of proteins, which is necessary in memory formation. But when this process is blocked, as in the brains of Alzheimer's patients, the effect on memory is disastrous.

Much of the research in the development of cognitive enhancers is focused on the activity of cyclic-AMP response element binding protein (CREB) in the hippocampus of the brain. CREB is a transcription factor thought to be important in memory and learning in organisms as diverse as Aplasia (a type of sea slug), Drosophila, and humans.

CREB is involved in the capacity for long-term memory through a phenomenon called long-term potentiation (LTP), which is thought to be important in learning and memory. LTP occurs when a large amount of neurotransmitter is released from one neuron to another, triggering a biochemical cascade that strengthens the connection (called a synapse) between the two neurons.

Evidence supports a model that the CREB pathway regulates memory by controlling the expression of proteins that promote synaptic plasticity. Plasticity is the ability of the brain to change the structure and function of synapses in response to cell signaling.

Drugs targeting this pathway may offer an effective way to reverse memory impairment in normal, age-related neurodegeneration, as well as in disease. The benefit of such treatments may be a wider therapeutic window and more general use since they target basic mechanisms in memory formation and are not limited to a specific pathology.

While many researchers are focusing on the hippocampus, others emphasize the fact that the brain is a heterogeneous structure with many parts involved in memory. The prefrontal cortex (PFC), for instance, is important in working memory such as intelligent thought, planning, and organization. The chemical needs of different parts of the brain are different, so drugs that may improve fixed memory for long-term storage in the hippocampus may at the same time impair dynamic updating of working memory in the prefrontal cortex.

The development of successful cognitive enhancers will have to consider the full complexity of the brain. In the meantime, an alliance of academic researchers is working on animal models to facilitate finding better gene targets in the search for memory enhancing drugs.

The Future
At least 40 potential cognitive enhancers are currently in clinical development. Many of the new compounds being scrutinized seek to improve the way recent memories are stored, transformed into long-term memories, and brought back into consciousness when needed.

Cognitive enhancers offer hope for millions whose current treatment options are bleak. On November 14, 2004, four scientists involved in research on cognitive enhancers met with the Neuro-degerative Diseases Discussion Group to discuss the feasibility of such drugs and the various strategies being pursued in their labs.

Vitamin E

- In *ONE* randomized, controlled study, Vitamin E showed some effectiveness in delaying progression
  - Study had 2000 IU/d
  - No longer advised

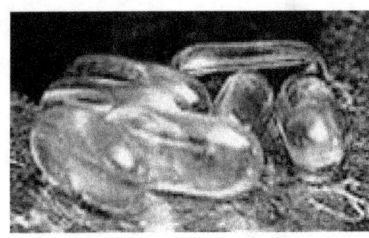

Last but not least there is one randomized placebo-controlled study that suggests Vitamin E had an effect similar to the cognitive enhancers in the delay of nursing home placement. The advantages of trying this option out are obvious, and very often we start both Vitamin E and Aricept together. It should be said that the study involved a mega-dose of Vitamin E---2000IU/day.

Source: (Kennard, 2005)

How Research into Vitamin E Shows Promise

In Alzheimer's, as in aging generally, there is an increase in free radical formation. Vitamin E is an antioxidant thought to protect neurons by reducing free radical formation and preventing cell injury. Free radicals occur as a result of a normal cell function called 'oxidative metabolism'. Free radicals are highly reactive. They attack other cells, damage cell walls, DNA, as well as metabolic processes.

Significant Research into Vitamin E

Research from the Alzheimer's Cooperative Society reported in 1997 their findings on the effectiveness of vitamin E and Selegiline. Focusing on functional loss, the results suggested both vitamin E and Selegiline delayed nursing home placement, death and disability but not cognitive functions (as scored in memory and thinking tests). The researchers found no differences between combined use of vitamin E and Selegiline or from groups of participants receiving the individual substances. Dosages used in the study were 10 mg of selegiline once daily and/or 1,000 IU of vitamin E twice daily.

Conclusion

Whilst this study is of great interest research is required that replicates their findings.

Further research is required that determines the effectiveness of treatment with these agents, in what combination and at what point in the different stages of Alzheimer's.

Appropriate therapeutic dosages of vitamin E needs to be established.

Side effects are possible with any drug. Selegiline in higher dosages can interact badly with some foods and drugs. People taking drugs like Warfarin should seek the expertise of their doctor. In general vitamin E is tolerated by most people without any problems.

Costs of the two agents mean that at the present time, and unless Selegiline is found to be a superior and more effective treatment, that Vitamin E is the agent of choice as it is much less expensive.

A review of the research, the Cochrane review has said that once adjustments are made for the study subjects (there were concerns that the study subjects were younger and therefore had less coexisting medical problems), that there is little evidence that vitamin E is of much use for people with Alzheimer's disease.

It is clear more research is required into the use of vitamin E.

Conclusions

- Prevalence of dementia will increase
- Brief screening tools exist
- Empirically validated treatments exist
- Consider the etiology
- Nonpharmacological interventions are also "treatments."
- Refer if necessary or if presentation atypical

Conclusions
- The prevalence of dementia will increase as the population ages.
- Brief cognitive screening tools exist and should be used to aid in earlier diagnosis.
- Epically validated treatments exist and may be more effective when used earlier in the disease course.
- The etiology of the dementia can influence treatment choice, even if when the dementia is due to some neurodegenerative disease process.

- Non-pharmacological interventions should also be considered treatments in their own right.
- Finally referral to a specialist may be helpful if the client's presentation is atypical in someway.

Works Cited

About.com Alzheimer's Disease. (n.d.). *Importance of Early Diagnosis in Alzheimer's Disease*. Retrieved Oct 2010, from http://alzheimers.about.com/od/diagnosisissues/a/early_diagnosis.htm

Alzheimer's Association. (n.d.). *OVERVIEW OF ALZHEIMER'S DISEASE*. Retrieved Apr 2010, from Alzheimer's Disease Information - Alzheimer's Association: http://www.alzpa.org/

Alzheimer's Disease: Causes, Symptoms, Treatment. (2010, Feb). *Cholinesterase inhibitors for Alzheimers disease patients*. Retrieved Nov 2010, from http://alzheimers-review.blogspot.com/2010/02/cholinesterase-inhibitors-for.html

Curtis, P. (2007, March 30). *Alzheimer's sufferers dying in drug 'scandal'*. Retrieved Apr 2009, from Guardian.co.uk: http://www.guardian.co.uk/society/2007/mar/30/health.medicineandhealth

Encyclopedia of Mental Disorders. (n.d.). *Wechsler adult intelligence scale*. Retrieved Feb 2010, from http://www.minddisorders.com/Py-Z/Wechsler-adult-intelligence-scale.html

Felthous, A. (2007). The International Handbook of Psychopathic Disorders and the Law. In A. Felthous, *The International Handbook of Psychopathic Disorders and the Law.* West Sussex, England: John Wiley & Sons Ltd.

Halim, N. (n.d.). *Cognitive Enhancers: The New Frontier in Treating Aging and Dementia*. Retrieved Oct 2010, from Cerebral Health: http://www.cerebralhealth.com/cognitiveenhancersfrontier.php

Kennard, C. (2005, Nov 13). *Vitamin E Treatments in Alzheimer's*. Retrieved Nov 2010, from About.com: Alzheimer's Disease: http://alzheimers.about.com/od/treatmentoptions/a/vitaminE.htm

Leutwyler, K. (2001, Aug). *Toward Early Diagnosis of Alzheimer's Disease*. Retrieved Oct 2010, from Scientific American: http://www.scientificamerican.com/article.cfm?id=toward-early-diagnosis-of

Martinon-Torres, G. (n.d.). *Trazodone for agitation in dementia*. Retrieved Nov 2010, from The Cochrane Collaboration: http://www2.cochrane.org/reviews/en/ab004990.html

National Institute on Aging. (n.d.). *Alzheimer's Disease Fact Sheet*. Retrieved Nov 2010, from http://www.nia.nih.gov/Alzheimers/Publications/adfact.htm

Wrongdiagnosis.com. (n.d.). *Systemic disorders*. Retrieved Nov 2010, from http://www.wrongdiagnosis.com/s/systemic_disorders/intro.htm

Chapter 6 - Other Dementia Syndromes

Not exhaustive, but other major types of dementia include:
- Vascular Dementia.
- Dementia with Lewy Bodies.
- Lewy Body vs. Parkinson's.
- Cortical Lewy Bodies.
- Frontotemporal dementias specifically Pick's Disease.

Interventions in the treatment of each will also be discussed.

Vascular Dementia

- Second most common form after AD

- One or more strokes, two or more cognitive functions affected

- Abrupt onset and stepwise course-- different from AD

- Aka "Binswanger's Disease," "lacunar state," or "multi-infarct dementia"

Source: (Alagiakrishnan, 2010)

The second most common form of dementia after Alzheimer's disease is vascular dementia. This form of dementia is caused by one or more strokes. The definition of the dementia is essentially the same as for any other, i.e., there should be memory impairment, and one other cognitive deficit associated with a significant decline in functioning. The onset is classically described as abrupt and the decline is classically stepwise, but this may be very difficult to determine. Other names for this syndrome have included Binswanger's Disease, a "lacunar" state, or multi infarct dementia.

Background

Vascular dementia is the second most common form of dementia after Alzheimer disease (AD). The condition is not a single disease; it is a group of syndromes relating to different vascular mechanisms. Vascular dementia is preventable; therefore, early detection and an accurate diagnosis are important. Clients who have had a stroke are at increased risk for vascular dementia. Recently, vascular lesions have been thought to play a role in AD.

As early as 1899, arteriosclerosis and senile dementia were described as different syndromes. In 1969, Mayer-Gross et al described this syndrome and reported that hypertension is the cause in approximately 50% of clients. In 1974, Hachinski et al coined the term multi-infarct dementia. In 1985, Loeb used the broader term vascular dementia. Recently, Bowler and Hachinski introduced a new term, vascular cognitive impairment.

Frequency
International

- Vascular dementia is the second most common cause of dementia in the United States and Europe, but it is the most common form in some parts of Asia.
- The prevalence rate of vascular dementia is 1.5% in Western countries and approximately 2.2% in Japan.
- In Japan, vascular dementia accounts for 50% of all dementias that occur in individuals older than 65 years.
- In Europe, vascular dementia and mixed dementia account for approximately 20% and 40% of cases, respectively.
- In Latin America, 15% of all dementias are vascular.
- In community-based studies in Australia, the prevalence rate for vascular and mixed dementia is 13% and 28%, respectively.
- The prevalence rate of dementia is 9 times higher in clients who have had a stroke than in controls. One year after a stroke, 25% of clients develop new-onset dementia. Within 4 years following a stroke, the relative risk of incident dementia is 5.5%.

Mortality/Morbidity

In clients with dementia who have had a stroke, the increase in mortality is significant. The 5-year survival rate is 39% for clients with vascular dementia compared with 75% for age-matched controls. Vascular dementia is associated with a higher mortality rate than AD, presumably because of the coexistence of other atherosclerotic diseases.

Sex

The prevalence of vascular dementia is higher in men than in women.

Age

Incidence increases with age.

Vascular Dementia
(DSM-IV - APA, 1994)
A. Multiple Cognitive Impairments
B. Deficits Impair Social/Occupational
C. Focal Neurological Signs and Symptoms or Laboratory Evidence indicating Cerebrovascular Disease Etiologically related to Deficits
D. Not Due to Delirium

Source: (Alagiakrishnan, 2010)

Treatment

Medical Care

The mainstay of management of vascular dementia is the prevention of new strokes. This includes administering antiplatelet drugs and controlling major vascular risk factors. Aspirin has also been found to slow the progression of vascular dementia.

Recent guidelines from the American Psychiatric Association provide both treatment principles and possible specific therapies.

Drug treatment is primarily used to prevent further worsening of vascular dementia by treating the underlying disease such as hypertension, hyperlipidemia, and diabetes mellitus. Antiplatelet agents are indicated.

Pentoxifylline and, to a more limited extent, ergoloid mesylates (Hydergine), may be useful for increasing cerebral blood flow. In the European Pentoxifylline Multi-Infarct Dementia Study, which is a double-blinded, placebo-controlled, multicenter study, treatment with pentoxifylline was found to be beneficial for clients with multi-infarct dementia. Significant improvement was observed in the scales used for assessing intellectual and cognitive function.

Neuroprotective drugs such as nimodipine, propentofylline, and posatirelin are currently under study and may be useful for vascular dementia.

Increasing evidence supports the involvement of the cholinergic system in vascular dementia, similar to that seen in Alzheimer dementia. However, no cholinesterase inhibitors have been approved to date for the treatment of vascular dementia, despite positive results in clinical trials with this medication.

The general management of dementia includes appropriate referral to community services, judgment and decision-making regarding legal and ethical issues (e.g., driving, competency, advance directives), and consideration of caregiver stress.

Diet
In the Rotterdam study, an increased risk of vascular dementia was associated with total fat intake, whereas fish consumption was inversely related to dementia.

Low levels of folate, vitamin B-6, and vitamin B-12 are associated with increased homocysteine levels, a risk factor for stroke.

Vascular Dementia

• Reserved for patients with clear evidence of stroke on imaging or physical exam
  – 10-40% of all dementia cases
  – 10-15% of AD cases are "mixed"
  – Treatment focused on risk factors
    • smoking
    • atrial fibrillation
    • diabetes
    • hypertension

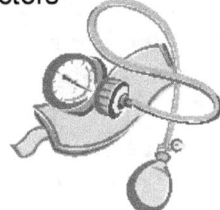

Source: (Alagiakrishnan, 2010)

The diagnosis of Vascular Dementia should be reserved for cases where there is some obvious neurological deficit on physical examination or where there is a clear finding on neuroimaging. VD accounts for 10-40% of all dementia cases. Because both VD and AD are common, you can also see "mixed dementias" where one client may have both disease processes.

The treatment of Vascular Dementia tends to be focused on risk factors that predispose to cerebrovascular illness. These would include atrial fibrillation, smoking, diabetes, hypertension etc.

Theoretically VD need not be as progressive as Alzheimer's disease. Families and clients can be informed of this to encourage compliance with treatment. However, if the client lives long enough, you cannot say that they are guaranteed NOT to get Alzheimer's disease as well.

Medico-legal Pitfalls
Dementia is a condition of impaired memory and cognition. Early in the course of vascular dementia, competence and capacity may be relatively intact. Clients may be able to manage their own affairs, provide consent for medical treatments, execute living

wills, or nominate a durable power of attorney for health care and finances.

As the dementia progresses, competency, and capacity are impaired. Sometimes, severe incapacitating dementia can occur before protective legal decisions are made. In such instances, the court may need to appoint a guardian, conservator, or trustee. The term trustee applies to a person appointed by law to execute a trust for the benefit of the beneficiary. A guardian or conservator is a person who has the legal power to take care of and/or manage the property of an incompetent person.

Special Concerns
Ethical issues must be considered on an individual basis, with consideration of clinical judgment and general ethical principles.

Frequently arising ethical issues and dilemmas in the care of individuals with vascular dementia are as follows:
- Dementia and driving.
- Consent for treatment and care.
- Physical and chemical restraints.
- Issues of end-of-life care, including artificial nutrition and hydration.

Dementia with Lewy Bodies

- High Incidence: 7-26%!

- Memory Impairment may come AFTER

- Visual hallucinations, delirium, parkinsonism

- Sensitive to neuroleptics

- Decline faster than AD?

Another Dementia syndrome is that of Dementia with Lewy Bodies or Lewy Body dementia. This dementia may have a higher incidence than previously thought…perhaps between 7-26%. The diagnosis of this disorder can be tricky. Because memory impairment may come after the onset of visual hallucinations, delirium, and parkinsonian symptoms.

These clients are very sensitive to neuroleptics which have been associated with an increased mortality. The decline can be faster than in Alzheimer's disease.

Source: (National Institute of Neurological Disorders and Stroke)
What is Dementia with Lewy Bodies?

Dementia with Lewy Dodies (DLB) is one of the most common types of progressive dementia. The central feature of DLB is progressive cognitive decline, combined with three additional defining features: (1) pronounced "fluctuations" in alertness and attention, such as frequent drowsiness, lethargy, lengthy periods of time spent staring into space, or disorganized speech; (2) recurrent visual hallucinations, and (3) parkinsonian motor symptoms, such as rigidity and the loss of spontaneous movement. People may also suffer from depression. The symptoms of DLB are caused by the build-up of Lewy Bodies – accumulated bits of alpha-synuclein protein -- inside the nuclei of neurons in areas of the brain that control particular aspects of memory and motor control. Researchers do not know exactly why alpha-synuclein accumulates into Lewy Bodies or how Lewy Bodies cause the symptoms of DLB, but they do know that alpha-synuclein accumulation is also linked to Parkinson's disease, multiple system atrophy, and several other disorders, which are referred to as the "synucleinopathies." The similarity of symptoms between DLB and Parkinson's disease, and between DLB and Alzheimer's disease, can often make it difficult for a doctor to make a definitive diagnosis. In addition, Lewy Bodies are often also found in the brains of people with Parkinson's and Alzheimer's diseases. These findings suggest that either DLB is related to these other causes of dementia or that an individual can have both diseases at the same time. DLB usually occurs sporadically, in people with no known family history of the disease. However, rare familial cases have occasionally been reported.

Is there any treatment?
There is no cure for DLB. Treatments are aimed at controlling the cognitive, psychiatric, and motor symptoms of the disorder. Acetyl cholinesterase inhibitors, such as donepezil and rivastigmine, are primarily used to treat the cognitive symptoms of DLB, but they may also be of some benefit in reducing the psychiatric and motor symptoms. Doctors tend to avoid prescribing antipsychotics for hallucinatory symptoms of DLB because of the risk that neuroleptic sensitivity could worsen the motor symptoms. Some individuals with DLB may benefit from the use of levodopa for their rigidity and loss of spontaneous movement.

What is the prognosis?
Like Alzheimer's disease and Parkinson's disease, DLB is a neurodegenerative disorder that results in progressive intellectual and functional deterioration. There are no known therapies to stop or slow the progression of DLB. Average survival after the time of diagnosis is similar to that in Alzheimer's disease, about 8 years, with progressively increasing disability.

Key symptoms are:

- Mild problems with recent memory, such as forgetting very recent events.

- Brief episodes of unexplained confusion and other behavioral or cognitive problems. The individual may become disoriented about the time or where he or she is; have trouble with speech, finding words or following a conversation, and experience visuospatial difficulty (such as finding one's way or working a jigsaw puzzle); and problems in thinking such as inattention, mental inflexibility, indecisiveness, lack of judgment and loss of insight.

- Fluctuation in the occurrence of these cognitive symptoms from moment to moment, hour to hour, day to day, or week to week. For example, the person may converse normally one day and be mute, unable to speak the next day — or even from one moment to the next. While this is often felt to be an important part of DLB, it may occur in other dementias and is sometimes it is very difficult to determine whether fluctuation truly occurs in a given client.

- Well-defined, vivid, visual hallucinations. In DLB's early stage, the person may even acknowledge and describe the hallucinations. Other types of hallucinations are less common but sometimes occur. These might be auditory ("hearing" sounds), olfactory ("tasting" something) or tactile ("feeling" something that isn't there).

- Movement (motor function) problems of Parkinsonism sometimes referred to as "extrapyramidal" signs. These symptoms often seem to start spontaneously and may include flexed posture, shuffling gait, reduced arm swing, limb stiffness, a tendency to fall, bradykinesia (slowness of movement), and tremor.

- Movement and motor problems occur in later stages for 70% of persons with DLB. But for 30% of DLB clients and more commonly those that are older, Parkinson's symptoms occur first, before dementia symptoms. In these individuals cognitive decline tends to start with depression or mild forgetfulness.

Lewy Body vs Parkinson's

- In DLB, Lewy Bodies are *cortical*
- In (idiopathic) Parkinson's Disease, Lewy Bodies in *substantia nigra*
- In PD, motor symptoms precede dementia *for years*
- In LBD motor symptoms more closely linked to memory problems

---

- Dementia with LB is not the same thing as the dementia associated with PD.
- Lewy Bodies are inclusion bodies found in the neuron that kill the cell.
- In dementia with lewy bodies, the lewy bodies are cortical.
- In idiopathic.

Source: ((TLC Senior Care)
Parkinson's disease the Lewy Bodies are in the substantia nigra. In Parkinson's disease motor symptoms precede the dementia for years. In Lewy Body dementia the motor symptoms are historically more closely linked to the memory problems.

Parkinson's, Alzheimer's, and Lewy Body Disease
Since Lewy Body Disease is commonly misdiagnosed for both
Parkinson's and Alzheimer's, it is helpful to understand how these
diseases overlap.

Some of the motor symptoms found in both Parkinson's and Lewy
Body Disease's clients include:
- Tremors.
- Muscle stiffness.
- Difficulties with balance.
- Shuffling gait.
- Stooped posture.
- Slow movements.
- Restless leg syndrome.

Some of the cognitive symptoms found in both Alzheimer's and
Lewy Body's clients include:
- Behavioral changes.
- Decreased judgment.
- Confusion and temporal/spatial disorientation.
- Difficulty following directions.
- Decreased ability to communicate.

Proactive Ways to Manage Lewy Body Disease

- **Become informed.** Learn as much as you can about Lewy
  Body Disease and how it is likely to affect you specifically,
  given your health history, age, and lifestyle.

- **Strengthen senses.** Have your doctor evaluate each of
  your five senses — sound, vision, touch, taste and smell —
  in order to identify and treat any abnormalities. Then ask
  about exercises to improve them. By challenging yourself
  to enhance your sense of sight, hearing, touch, taste, and
  smell, you will boost both your mental and physical
  capabilities.

- **Manage symptoms with behavioral changes.** One example of symptom management in LBD involves low blood pressure (hypotension), a common Lewy Body Disease symptom that can lead to falls. To help stabilize your blood pressure and minimize the risk of fall-related injuries, be sure to stay well hydrated, exercise, get adequate sodium (salt) in your diet, avoid prolonged bed rest, and stand up slowly.

- **Choose medications wisely.** The potential benefits of any medication need to be carefully balanced with possible side effects that may occur. In people with Lewy Body Disease, the treatments for hallucinations, delusions, and behavioral disturbance tend to make the Parkinson's symptoms worse; and treating the Parkinson's symptoms can make the delusions and behavior problems worse. However, depression and sleep disorders can and should be treated with medications that the client can safely tolerate.

Parkinson's disease is a progressive disorder of the central nervous system that affects more than 1.5 million people in the United States. The main features of Parkinson's disease are slowness of movements, compromise of balance, muscle rigidity, and tremor. The disease is thought to be caused by low levels of a chemical called dopamine, which activates cells in our brains that let us move.

Symptoms of Parkinson's Disease
There are primary and secondary symptoms of Parkinson's disease. Not everyone with the disease experiences all of the symptoms and the progression of the disease is different from person to person. Most people who get Parkinson's are over 60, but recently there have been more identified cases in younger men and women.

Most of the symptoms of the disease involve disruption of motor functions (muscle and movement). However, lack of energy, mood and memory changes, and pain can also occur as part of the disease.

Primary symptoms of Parkinson's disease:
- Bradykinesia – slowness in voluntary movement such as standing up, walking, and sitting down. This happens because of delayed transmission signals from the brain to the muscles. This may lead to difficulty initiating walking, but when more severe can cause "freezing episodes" once walking has begun.
- Tremors – often occur in the hands, fingers, forearms, foot, mouth, or chin. Typically, tremors take place when the limbs are at rest as opposed to when there is movement.
- Rigidity – otherwise known as stiff muscles, often produce muscle pain that is increased during movement.
- Poor balance – happens because of the loss of reflexes that help posture. This causes unsteady balance, which oftentimes leads to falls.

Secondary symptoms of Parkinson's disease:
- Constipation.
- Difficulty swallowing.
- Choking, coughing, or drooling.
- Excessive salivation.
- Excessive sweating.
- Loss of bowel and/or bladder control.
- Loss of intellectual capacity.
- Anxiety, depression, isolation.
- Scaling, dry skin on the face or scalp.
- Slow response to questions.
- Small cramped handwriting.
- Soft, whispery voice.

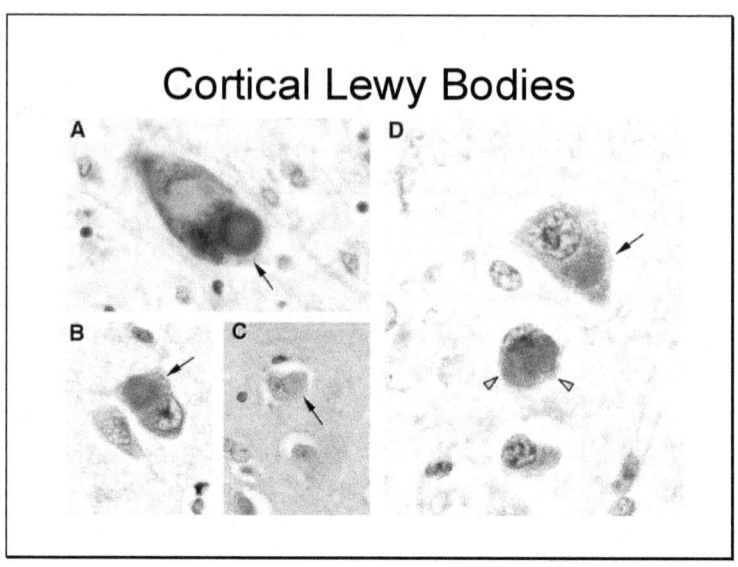

Cortical Lewy Bodies

Here are some pictures of cortical Lewy Bodies found at autopsy in a client with Lewy Body Dementia.

Source: (Papka, 1998)

A, Typical appearance of a mature Lewy body (***arrow***) in a pigmented neuron of the substantia nigra.

B, Lewy Bodies (***arrow***) typically are more indistinct in cortical neurons but are still readily identified on ubiquitin immunostains

C, Cortical Lewy Bodies (***arrow***)

D, Making a distinction between globose tangles (***arrowheads***)— fibrillar accumulations that fill the cytoplasm of small, round neurons—and Lewy Bodies (***arrow***)—which form discrete, rounded homogeneous intracytoplasmic inclusions—is critical for accurate evaluation of Alzheimer's disease stage or concurrent Parkinson's disease pathology

What are Lewy Bodies?
In 1912, while Frederick Lewy was examining the brains of people with Parkinson's disease, he discovered irregularities in the cells in

the mid-brain region. These abnormal structures (microscopic protein deposits found in deteriorating nerve cells) became known as Lewy Bodies. Since that time, the presence of Lewy Bodies in the mid-brain has been recognized as a hallmark of Parkinson's disease. In the 1960s, researchers found Lewy Bodies in the cortex (the outer layer of gray matter) of the brains of some people who had dementia. Lewy Bodies in the cortex are known as cortical Lewy Bodies or diffuse Lewy Bodies. (That is why Lewy body disease is sometimes called cortical Lewy body disease or diffuse Lewy body disease.) Cortical Lewy Bodies were thought to be rare, until the 1980s when improved methodologies showed that Lewy body disease was more common than previously realized.

People with Lewy body disease have Lewy Bodies in the mid-brain region (like those with Parkinson's disease) and in the cortex of the brain. It has believed that they usually also have the "plaques and tangles" of the brain that characterize Alzheimer's disease. Conversely, it is believed that many people with Alzheimer's disease also have cortical Lewy Bodies. Because of the overlap, it is likely that many people with Lewy body disease are misdiagnosed (at least initially) as having either Parkinson's disease or Alzheimer's disease. A big factor in the misdiagnosis might be that Lewy body disease is relatively unknown.

Frontotemporal

- Pick's Disease is type of frontotemporal dementia
  - Personality changes, lower inhibition, executive dysfunction
  - Memory impairment
  - FT atrophy on brain imaging. Assymetric?

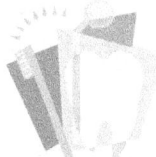

Frontotemporal dementias represent another category of neurodegenerative dementias. Pick's Disease is one of the frontal-temporal dementias. The presentation of clients with this type of dementia is characterized by personality changes, lowered inhibition of behaviors, affect, and executive functioning. Again, in order for it to warrant the diagnosis of dementia, some memory impairment must be present as well.

It is possible to see localized atrophy on brain imaging in client's with this type of dementia. That is, the atrophy in the frontal or temporal lobes can be more profound than in other areas of brain. The atrophy can even be asymmetric.

Definition
Frontotemporal dementia (frontotemporal lobar degeneration) is an umbrella term for a diverse group of uncommon disorders that primarily affect the frontal and temporal lobes of the brain — the areas generally associated with personality, behavior, and language.

In frontotemporal dementia, portions of these lobes atrophy, or shrink. Signs and symptoms vary, depending upon the portion of the brain affected. Some people with frontotemporal dementia undergo dramatic changes in their personality and become socially inappropriate, impulsive or emotionally blunted, while others lose the ability to use and understand language.

Frontotemporal dementia is often misdiagnosed as a psychiatric problem or as Alzheimer's disease. But frontotemporal dementia tends to occur at a younger age than does Alzheimer's disease, typically between the ages of 40 and 70.

Symptoms
Identifying precisely which diseases fall into the category of frontotemporal dementia presents a particular challenge to scientists. The signs and symptoms may vary greatly from one individual to the next. Researchers have identified several clusters of symptoms that tend to occur together and be dominant in

subgroups of people with the disorder. More than one symptom cluster may be apparent in the same person.

Behavioral Changes
The most common signs and symptoms of frontotemporal dementia involve extreme changes in behavior and personality. These include:
- Increasingly inappropriate actions.
- Euphoria.
- Lack of judgment and inhibition.
- Apathy.
- Repetitive compulsive behavior.
- A decline in personal hygiene.
- Lack of awareness of thinking or behavioral changes.

Speech and Language Problems
Some subtypes of frontotemporal dementia are marked by the impairment or loss of speech and linguistic abilities. For example, primary progressive aphasia is characterized by an increasing difficulty in using and understanding written and spoken language. People with another subtype, semantic dementia, utter grammatically correct speech that has no relevance to the conversation at hand.

Movement Disorders
Rarer subtypes of frontotemporal dementia are characterized by problems with movement, similar to those associated with Parkinson's disease or amyotrophic lateral sclerosis (ALS) — which is also often called Lou Gehrig's disease. Movement-related signs and symptoms may include:
- Tremor.
- Rigidity.
- Muscle spasms.
- Poor coordination.
- Difficulty swallowing.
- Muscle weakness.

Treatments and Drugs

There is no cure for frontotemporal dementia and no effective way to slow its progression. Treatment relies on managing the symptoms.

Medications

Antidepressants. Some types of antidepressants, such as trazodone, may reduce the behavioral problems associated with frontotemporal dementia. Selective serotonin reuptake inhibitors (SSRIs) have also been effective in some cases, although study results have been mixed.

Antipsychotics. Although antipsychotic drugs are sometimes used to combat the behavioral problems of frontotemporal dementia, side effects can include an increased risk of mortality in older people.

Therapy

People experiencing language difficulties may benefit from speech therapy, to learn alternate strategies for communication

Lifestyle and Home Remedies

In some cases, caregivers can reduce behavior problems by changing the way they interact with people who have dementia. Examples include:

- Avoiding events or activities that trigger the behavior.
- Anticipating needs and alleviating them promptly.
- Maintaining a calm environment.

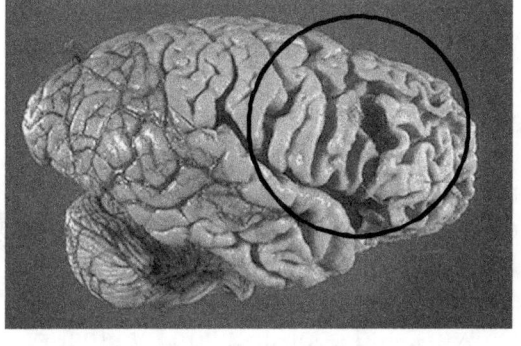

Pick's Disease aka "Walnut Brain"

This is a gross brain specimen from an individual with Pick's disease.

As you can see the atrophy is most pronounced in the frontal area of the brain although it does exist elsewhere too. The pathologists' jargon for this type of atrophy is "Walnut Brain." Pick's Disease causes a slow shrinking of brain cells due to excess protein build-up. Clients initially exhibit marked personality and behavioral changes, and a decline in the ability to speak coherently.

While up to seven million Americans may be afflicted with FTDs, Pick's Disease accounts for just five percent of all progressive dementias. It is frequently misdiagnosed in the early stages as depression, mental illness, or Alzheimer's disease, because of the manner in which symptoms initially appear.

Source: (HelpGuide.org)
What is Pick's Disease?
According to Arnold Pick, who first described the disease in 1892, Pick's Disease causes an irreversible decline in a person's functioning over a period of years. Although it is commonly confused with the much more prevalent Alzheimer's disease, Pick's Disease is a rare disorder that causes the frontal and temporal lobes

of the brain, which control speech and personality, to slowly atrophy. It is therefore classified as a "frontotemporal dementia", or FTD.

According to the National Institute of Neurological Disorders and Stroke, the following conditions are currently grouped together as frontotemporal dementias:

Causes and Risk Factors of Pick's Disease
Like Huntington's disease and Lewy Body Disease, Pick's Disease is the result of a build-up of protein in the affected areas of the brain. The accumulation of abnormal brain cells, known as Pick's bodies, eventually leads to changes in character, socially inappropriate behavior, and poor decision making, progressing to a severe impairment in intellect, memory, and speech.

Pick's Disease usually strikes adults between the ages of 40 and 60, and is slightly more common in women than in men. While the cause is still unknown, there is a strong genetic component: FTDs tend to run in families, and approximately 40% of Pick's Disease cases are believed to be hereditary.

Signs and Symptoms of Pick's Disease
Because the frontal lobes affect behavior and emotional response, people with Pick's Disease will usually show signs of changes in personality before they manifest evidence of dementia. This may begin as impulsiveness or a lack of inhibition. While the progression of symptoms in Pick's Disease is fortunately slow, symptoms do worsen over time.
The following symptoms are typical of clients with Pick's Disease. More severe symptoms will appear in later stages of the illness.

Behavioral Changes
- Impulsivity.
- Obsessive/compulsiveness (for example, overeating or only eating one type of food).
- Drinking alcohol to excess (when this was not previously a problem).
- Rudeness or impatience, leading to aggression.

- Poor judgment.
- Inability to function or interact in social situations.
- Inability to hold a job.
- Lack of attention to personal hygiene.
- Sexual exhibitionism or promiscuity.
- Withdrawal or seclusion.

Emotional Changes
- Abrupt mood changes.
- Lack of warmth, concern, or empathy.
- Indifference to events or to one's environment.
- Easily distracted; difficulty maintaining a line of thought.
- Unaware of the changes in behavior.
- Decreased interest in activities of daily living.

Language Changes
- Reduced quality of speech: shrinking vocabulary, difficulty finding a word.
- Difficulty speaking or understanding speech (aphasia).
- Repeating words others say (echolalia).
- Weak, uncoordinated speech sounds.
- Decreased ability to read or write.
- Complete loss of speech (mute).

Neurological and Physical Problems
- Increased muscle rigidity or stiffness.
- Difficulty moving about.
- Lack of coordination.
- General weakness.
- Memory loss.
- Urinary incontinence.
- Managing Pick's Disease.

Focusing on the positive aspects of dealing with a terminal disease might seem like an exercise in futility, and yet, there can be unexpected bright spots for clients with Pick's Disease. For instance, at the University of California/San Francisco Medical Center's Memory and Aging Center, doctors discovered a small group of frontotemporal dementia clients who developed new creative skills in music and art. The artistic talents emerged when the brain cell loss occurred predominantly in the left frontal lobe, which controls functions such as language.

As the ability to communicate through words declined, these clients' brains somehow accessed other realms of self-expression. So exploring and encouraging the development of latent skills is one way in which Pick's Disease clients can maintain their quality of life and possibly slow the progress of mental deterioration.

In addition, consider the following steps to help manage the symptoms of Pick's Disease:
- Sensory function aids, such as eyeglasses, hearing aids, etc.
- Behavior modification that rewards positive behaviors.
- Speech therapy and/or occupational therapy.

Medication to control behaviors that can be dangerous to oneself or others. Antidepressants known as selective serotonin reuptake inhibitors (SSRIs) may offer some relief from apathy and depression and help reduce food cravings, loss of impulse control and compulsive activity

---

Frontotemporal (Pick's)

- "Pre-senile" in onset: 50-60
- More progressive and rapidly deteriorating than AD
- Final diagnosis also autopsy-based

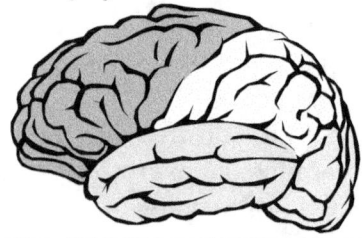

Source (HelpGuide.org)

Other things to remember about Frontotemporal Dementias include that they tend to be "presenile" in onset, that is, the typical age of onset is between 50 and 60 years of age.

The ultimate diagnosis is made at autopsy…these dementias also may have characteristic inclusion bodies.

Five Distinguishing Characteristics of Pick's Disease
- Onset before age 65.
- Initial personality changes.
- Loss of normal controls, e.g., gluttony, hyper sexuality.
- Lack of inhibition.
- Roaming behavior.

Works Cited

Alagiakrishnan, K. (2010, Oct 29). *Vascular Dementia*. Retrieved Nov 2010, from emedicine WebMD: http://emedicine.medscape.com/article/292105-overview

HelpGuide.org. (n.d.). *Pick's Disease: Signs, Symptoms, Treatment, and Suppport*. Retrieved Nov 2010, from HelpGuide: http://www.helpguide.org/elder/picks_disease.htm

National Institute of Neurological Disorders and Stroke. (n.d.). *NINDS Dementia With Lewy Bodies Information Page*. Retrieved Oct 2010, from http://www.ninds.nih.gov/disorders/dementiawithlewybodies/dementiawithlewybodies.htm

Papka, M. (1998, Aug). *A Review of Lewy Body Disease, an Emerging Concept of Cortical Dementia*. Retrieved Nov 2010, from Neuropsychiatry & Clinical Neurosciences: http://neuro.psychiatryonline.org/cgi/content/full/10/3/267

TLC Senior Care. (n.d.). *Lewy Body Disease: Signs, Symptoms and Treatment*. Retrieved Nove 2010, from TLC Senior Care: http://www.tlcseniorcare.com/49.html?new_sess=1

Weder, N. (2007, June). *Frontotemporal Dementias: A Review*. Retrieved Nov 2010, from Annals of General Psychiatry: http://www.annals-general-psychiatry.com/content/6/1/15

Chapter 7 - Helpful Approaches

Inclusion & Pacing

- Always include the client
  - Include them in conversations *about* them
- Don't rush
  - Slow down your overall pacing
    - Speak slowly (within reason)
    - Shhhhh….wait for a reply (within reason)

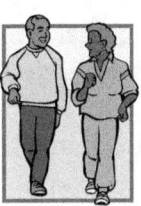

By including the client, you create:
- Shared responsibility.
- Greater buy in.
- Sense of purpose.

Do not rush:
- Processing speeds are slower.
- Two ears and one mouth.
- Allow silence, this is time for everyone to process.
- Silence is a sign of respect and confidence.
- Provide reassurance – particularly if the person can no longer recognize you.
- Play soft music in the background.
- Introduce a familiar physical object or activity.
- Post a daily schedule, and point to it when moving to the next item on the agenda.
- Adhere to the schedule.
- Use timers to remind the person of plans or activities.

- Try some of the adaptations suggested above under the section titled Memory and other cognitive functions .

Communicating with Dementia

By practicing these tips when talking with a person with Alzheimer's disease or a related dementia, both the care giver and the other person should experience more cooperation and less frustration. Never talk about the person as if he/she is not there. Show respect in all words and actions and achieve better understanding.

To gain person's attention:
- Look eye to eye.
- Speak the person's preferred name first, before beginning message.

To deliver message:
- Use simple adult words.
- Speak slowly and clearly.
- Do not shout - lower the pitch of your voice if you are female.
- Give one message at a time.

Listen for response:
- Allow time for response.
- Repeat the question, using the same words.
- Help person put words together.
- Validate the meaning of the response.
- Watch body language. How does the person feel?

Ask answerable questions:
- Limit choices - too many can be confusing.
- *Do not offer choices if there are none.*
- Ask uncomplicated questions, one at a time.
- In general, questions can put the person "on the spot" - use sparingly.

Use non-confronting, non-controlling statements:
- Agree first and then limit your response.
- Do not argue, but instead attempt to change the subject.
- Identify feelings rather than argue facts.
- Ignore repetitive statements if they are not emotionally charged.
- Ask for cooperation and help.

Reassure and calm:
- Use body language (gestures) to explain statements.
- Write a simple note.
- Tell the person that everything is going according to plan.
- Events measure time: "Before lunch" or "After lunch" rather than "In an hour."

Source: (Cummings)

As a person's dementia progresses, the ability, skills, and memory needed to communicate with others decreases. This is due to the increased damage to the brain. As the disease works its way through the brain, more of the lobes of the brain are affected. These various lobes control certain functions or behaviors in each person.

Two of these lobes, the frontal and the temporal contain much of the skills and memory needed for communication. But these lobes are also greatly affected by the disease process. These lobes shrink, fill with cerebrospinal fluid, or pieces of them disappear altogether. As the frontal lobes (short-term and long-term memory, speech, personality, impulse control, judgment, rational thought, attention, cognition and imagination) and the temporal lobes (language, hearing and smell) are damaged and eventually destroyed, memory and language skills are destroyed as well.

To continue to be able to communicate with our loved ones, we must alter our method of communication to allow them the best way to understand us. These are seven rules to remember when communicating with persons with dementia. Remember to prepare to communicate, no chewing gum, etc. Relax; don't cover your mouth while talking. Monitor your non-verbal communication like annoyance, frustration, impatience, or quick movements. Slow down, use shorter sentences, prepare to repeat information and think out of the box. Use an eraser board for example and write messages to facilitate communication. (Black ink on white board is recommended, we see it better.) Encourage eyeglasses and hearing aids, if needed. Persons who are older also hear and better understand a deeper tone of voice, so be certain to lower the pitch of your voice.

1. Always address the elder as an adult. Avoid baby talk or patronizing communication. Too often, loving caregivers fall into the habit of speaking to impaired adults as though they were children. Speaking with an exaggerated intonation or slow rate, overly simplified sentences, a higher pitched voice or referring to the person by pet names should be avoided.

   Non-familial caregivers should not refer to persons as "Momma" or "Poppa" or "Boyfriend" etc., as this is disrespectful and confusing to the person with the disease. Any tone, statement or gesture that can be perceived as a lack of respect can lead to resistance, so be aware some things are hardwired in the brain and are not lost until the end of the disease.

2. Keep communication conversational, not inquisitional. Have you ever been at a party of business function and a stranger asks, "Do you remember me? "How did that make you feel? Folks with dementia suffer the same emotions when well-meaning family and friends "quiz" them when starting a conversation. Questions like this put a person on the defensive and increases confusion.

   Instead try this approach: "Hi Aunt Betty. I'm Suzy and I'm your big sister Mary's oldest daughter. I used to come and stay with you during the summer and we would make cookies and bake pies. I always loved staying at your house in the country and feeding your chickens."

   This greeting gives the person a lot of information to work with including your name, your relation, and some long-term memories to start clues for conversation. Remember short-term memory is affected first and long-term memories stay intact and viable for a long time. Make each conversation successful! Knowing a person's background always improves a better conversation, so use it!

3. Always presume the person can hear or may understand the conversation. Even very advanced dementia patients can still tell when the conversation is about them. Do not talk "around" the person, but keep him or her a part of the conversation. Be polite, explain you are now discussing him or her with the caregiver and ask for permission to do so.

   Paranoia can already be a part of this person's world due to the inability to utilize the brain to understand the environment, i.e., hearing, sight, smell, touch, language, etc. So don't do social interactions that increase this behavior. Remember parts of social behavior are still functional and almost hardwired into the long-term memory of the brain. Many of us would become upset if we thought others were talking about us behind our backs.

4. Provide descriptive cues as well as accurate cues. Alert the person you are there and would like to talk or interact. A touch on the shoulder or hand, a handshake and eye contact help start the process. Now prepare to provide adequate information for this person.

Instead of "Here you are," and giving the person a glass of fluid and then walking away, try to give more information and instruction. A better approach would be "Mary, I brought you the glass of orange juice you wanted. You can drink it now."

This approach clued her to what is happening and what she is expected to do. She was addressed by name, the object was identified as a glass of orange juice and finally, she received a verbal clue the item was for her to drink. When you use this type of statement, the person is provided with a great deal of information as well of a social interaction that is more complex.

5. Provide as many clues and cues as possible for the person to alert him or her to the event. Touch, tell, show, invite or offer assistance. For example, as the disease progresses the person has a harder time recognizing physical clues, like the need to empty his or her bladder.

Simply asking "Do you need to go to the bathroom?" can result in a negative response of "No," followed a short time later with an accident. A method utilizing clues and cues would be to take the person by the hand and lead her to the bathroom and show her the commode. This type of cueing can prompt the person to realize her bladder is full.

6. Simplify tasks and break them down into achievable parts. Again use cues and clues. Don't just tell a person to get dressed to point to a shirt to wear. Minutes later you may find the person standing with the shirt and not a clue as to what to do or to the shirt's purpose.

Instead, tell her the steps involved. You can even help cue her by starting with putting an arm in the shirt, etc. Each individual situation calls for different cueing. Your experience will tell you what is involved with your elder.

7. Eliminate competing stimulation. Start with the right environment. Turn off the television and radio, face the person,

and speak clearly and distinctly. Maintain the social roles of conversation and encourage talking and listening with a variety of contexts and topics.

Other tips include "invite" the elder to participate rather than ordering or informing him now it's time to do such-and-such. Check to be certain of the person's comfort level with touch. Some people don't want to be touched by strangers and if the person doesn't recognize her family anymore, this can cause some conflict and pain for the family. Also, don't touch belongings without permission, as this can be misinterpreted. For example, you may pick up a photo off the mantle to discuss it with the person, but the person may think you are trying to take the photo or are invading her privacy. Watch and observe the behavior to determine how your moves are being interpreted.

Do not jump from topic to topic. Use a familiar vocabulary, preferably with nouns and not pronouns. Use gestures, pointing and pantomime to supplement the conversation.

Smile, show positive emotions and attitudes. The last thing the loved one needs is to see how depressed or stressed out you are about your life, but on the other hand…key into the emotion of the moment. If the person you are engaging is in an emotional fixation of some sort, try to relate to what they are feeling and address their fears and concerns.

Relax

- A hurried/anxious approach can cause anxiety or concern for people with dementia
- Don't startle them - come up from behind them and start talking
- Be present - focus on what you're doing

- Stay calm, even when they are not.
- Role model perfect behavior.
- Be aware their hearing is not what it used to be, nor is their peripheral awareness.
- Give them your full attention; it will make communication much more effective and a lot less frustrating.
- Provide new or more activities and things to do.
- Increase the variety of activities provided to include the different senses (e.g., particularly things that can be touched).
- Provide opportunities for more involvement in day-to-day activities (e.g., safe aspects of meal preparation, clean-up).
- Provide more social opportunities.

Give Them Space

– Stand with them not over them
– Be at eye level and slightly to one side
– "Hi, I'm (Name) - it's nice to see you"
– Avoid "do you remember…" they may not

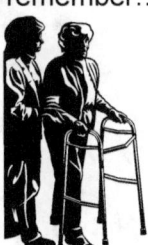

- Use of labels or pictures on cupboards to show content (e.g., coffee cup).
- Pasting familiar signs or images on doors to identify room function (e.g., toilet sign, picture of a bed).
- Creating a "memory box" that contains small personal items that can trigger meaningful conversation (e.g., pictures of family members, pets or possessions).

- Setting and maintaining the same daily schedule to provide a sense of control over the environment; posting the schedule on a picture board may also reduce often repeated questions.
- Prominently displaying clocks and calendars.
- Posting a list of favorite television programs with their times and channels near the TV to increase autonomy and decrease repetitive questions.
- Setting-up computer function keys, with meaningful stick-on labels, to facilitate easy Internet and e-mail connections.
- Using Velcro fasteners on clothing instead of buttons.

Humor and Gentle Enthusiasm

– Infectious and rapport building
– Avoid biting sarcasm or other forms of humor that may be mistaken for ridicule
– Be gently enthusiastic
  • Avoid "cheerleader" approach
    – Can cause stress or anxiety

Happiness Is 'Infectious' In Network of Friends: Collective -- Not Just Individual -- Phenomenon

Source: Science Daily (Dec. 5, 2008)
If you are happy and you know it, thank your friends—and their friends. And while you are at it, their friends' friends. But if you are sad, hold the blame. Researchers from Harvard Medical School and the University of California, San Diego have found that "happiness" is not the result solely of a cloistered journey filled with individually tailored self-help techniques. Happiness is also a

collective phenomenon that spreads through social networks like an emotional contagion.

In a study that looked at the happiness of nearly 5000 individuals over a period of twenty years, researchers found that when an individual becomes happy, the network effect can be measured up to three degrees. One person's happiness triggers a chain reaction that benefits not only their friends, but also their friends' friends, and their friends' friends' friends. The effect lasts for up to one year.

The flip side, interestingly, is not the case: Sadness does not spread through social networks as robustly as happiness. Happiness appears to love company more so than misery.

"We've found that your emotional state may depend on the emotional experiences of people you don't even know, who are two to three degrees removed from you," says Harvard Medical School professor Nicholas Christakis, who, along with James Fowler from the University of California, San Diego co-authored this study. "And the effect isn't just fleeting."

For over two years now, Christakis and Fowler have been mining data from the Framingham Heart Study (an ongoing cardiovascular study begun in 1948), reconstructing the social fabric in which individuals are enmeshed, and analyzing the relationship between social networks and health. The researchers uncovered a treasure trove of data from archived, handwritten administrative tracking sheets dating back to 1971. All family changes for each study participant, such as birth, marriage, death, and divorce, were recorded. In addition, participants had also listed contact information for their closest friends, coworkers, and neighbors. Coincidentally, many of these friends were also study participants. Focusing on 4,739 individuals, Christakis and Fowler observed over 50,000 social and family ties and analyzed the spread of happiness throughout this group.

Using the Center for Epidemiological Studies Depression Index (a standard metric) that study participants completed, the researchers found that when an individual becomes happy, a friend living within a mile experiences a 25 percent increased chance of becoming happy. A co-resident spouse experiences an 8 percent increased chance, siblings living within one mile have a 14 percent increased chance, and for next door neighbors, 34 percent.

But the real surprise came with indirect relationships. Again, while an individual becoming happy increases his friend's chances, a friend of that friend experiences a nearly 10 percent chance of increased happiness, and a friend of *that* friend has a 5.6 percent increased chance—a three-degree cascade.

"We've found that while all people are roughly six degrees separated from each other, our ability to influence others appears to stretch to only three degrees," says Christakis. "It's the difference between the structure and function of social networks."

These effects are limited by both time and space. The closer a friend lives to you, the stronger the emotional contagion. But as distance increases, the effect dissipates. This explains why next door neighbors have an effect, but not neighbors who live around the block. In addition, the happiness effect appears to wear off after roughly one year. "So the spread of happiness is constrained by time and geography," observes Christakis, who is also a professor of sociology in the Harvard Faculty of Arts and Sciences. "It can't just happen at any time, any place."

They also found that, contrary to what your parents taught you, popularity *does* lead to happiness. People in the center of their network clusters are the most likely people to become happy, odds that increase to the extent that the people surrounding them also have lots of friends. However, becoming happy does not help migrate a person from the network fringe to the center. Happiness spreads through the network without altering its structure.

"Imagine an aerial view of a backyard party," Fowler explains. "You'll see people in clusters at the center, and others on the outskirts. The happiest people tend to be the ones in the center. But someone on the fringe, who suddenly becomes happy, say through a particular exchange, does not suddenly move into the center of the group. He simply stays where he is—only now he has a far more satisfying sense of well-being. Happiness works not by changing where you're located in the network; it simply spreads through the network."

Fowler also points out that these findings give us an interesting perspective for this holiday season, which arrives smack in the middle of some pretty gloomy economic times. Examination of this dataset shows that having $5,000 extra increased a person's chances of becoming happier by about 2 percent. But that the same data also show, as Fowler notes, that "Someone you don't know and have never met—the friend of a friend of a friend—can have a greater influence than hundreds of bills in your pocket."

This is the third major network analysis by Christakis and Fowler that shows how our health is affected by our social context. The two previous studies, both published in the New England Journal of Medicine, described the social network effects in obesity and smoking cessation.

The research was funded by the National Institutes of Health/National Institute on Aging, a Pioneer Grant from the Robert Wood Johnson Foundation, and a contract from the National Heart, Lung, and Blood Institute to the Framingham Heart Study.

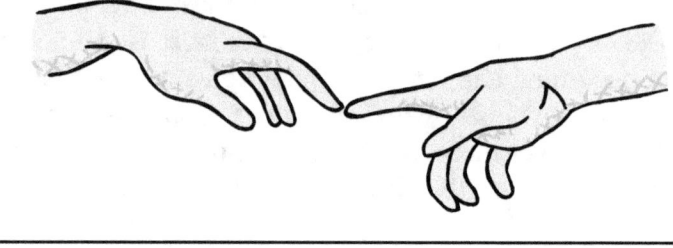

How The Power Of Touch Reduces Pain And Even Fights Disease
Source: (Dobson, 2006)
By Roger Dobson

When Jim Coan scanned the brains of married women in pain, he spotted changes that may help to shed light on an age-old mystery. As soon as the women touched the hands of their husbands, there was an instant drop in activity in the areas of the brains involved in fear, danger, and threat. The women, who had been exposed to experimental pain while they were scanned, were calmer and less stressed, and a similar, but smaller, effect was triggered by the touch of strangers.

Touch, a key component of traditional healing, is being increasingly studied in mainstream medicine, with some trials showing symptom benefits in a number of areas, from asthma and high blood pressure to migraine and childhood diabetes. Other research findings hint that not only does touch lower stress levels, but that it can boost the immune system and halt or slow the progress of disease.

Cincinnati Children's Hospital is one of a number of leading health centers in the US that now uses healing touch therapy. "Research has demonstrated that clients who receive healing touch experience accelerated wound healing and relaxation, pain relief and general comfort," said a spokesman.

Some believe the power of touch is all down to the placebo effect. "If you touch your partner they feel relaxed, but if someone else touches they may not feel as relaxed," said Professor Edward Ernst, a professor of complementary medicine at the University of Exeter. "That is very much mind over matter. It has nothing to with the sensations of being touched; it is the expectation and the context of the intervention, rather than the specific effect of that intervention."

While touch is used extensively for stress and anxiety and in palliative care, research is now increasingly focusing on whether it can impede the progress of a number of diseases, including depression and cancer.

Wounds took a day longer to heal when the client had been involved in an argument with a loved one, and that in married couples who did not get on, wound healing took two days longer. "Wounds in the couples who were hostile healed at only 60 per cent of the rate of couples with low levels of hostility," said Dr Janice Kiecolt-Glaser.

That finding, plus those of Dr Coan, may explain why the touch of a loved one can be therapeutic. But they do not explain why the touch of practitioners and strangers can have a similar effect. At DePauw University in Indiana, Dr Matthew Hertenstein may have found an answer. He has discovered that touch communicates emotions. When people were touched by a stranger they could not see, who had been instructed to try to communicate a particular emotion, they were able to tell the emotional state of the other person with great accuracy.

The findings show that people can communicate several distinct emotions through touch alone, including anger, fear, disgust, love, gratitude, and sympathy. Accuracy rates ranged from 48 per cent to 83 per cent, comparable with those found in studies of emotions shown in faces and voices. "The evidence indicates that humans can communicate several distinct emotions through touch," said Dr. Hertenstein. "Our study is the first to provide rigorous evidence showing that humans can reliably signal love, gratitude, and sympathy with touch. These findings raise the interesting possibility that touch may convey more positive emotions than the face."

How Hugs Can Heal
- Hugging your partner could lower his or her blood pressure.
- Researchers have found that in younger women, the more hugs they get, the lower, and their blood pressure.
- Researchers at the University of North Carolina who investigated 69 pre-menopausal women showed that those who had the most hugs had a reduced heart rate.
- Exactly what could be responsible is not clear, but the psychiatrists who carried out the work also found that blood levels of the hormone oxytocin were much higher in the women who were hugged the most.
- Other research finds that oxytocin is released during social contact and that it is associated with social bonding, while a study at Ohio State University shows that when it is put into wounds in animals, the injuries heal much more quickly.

Our need for human contact is necessary. Babies who are not touched fail to grow normally. Children, who are not lovingly touched often, grow up to be more physically violent. And that is a shame because our society is starting to become a "hands to ourselves" environment.

Here are a few beginning tips:

- Start by kissing friends hello on the cheek. If that makes you uncomfortable, try hugs. A good hug is a quick, anti-stress remedy, as spiritually healing as hours of meditation.

The person you are hugging has the power, with their touch, to free you from the tyranny of your restless mind.

- Begin with a friendly pat on a person's back. Walk arm and arm with a friend. When talking to someone, gently touch his or her arm or hand during the conversation. Small touches can go a long way to making a person's day.

- Rub your husband/partner's back for 30 minutes, and then insist on receiving one in turn.

- Yoga, running, swimming. Any exercise that stimulates your skin and has you pounding the ground is beneficial. Remember, touching* is often just as gratifying as being touched!

*Note: Concerns about sexual harassment have made touching a "touchy" issue. Just follow a few guidelines when touching:
- Stay away from body parts like buttocks, stomach, chest, and areas below the belt. Especially when hugging or touching other people's children.
- Men tend to be standoffish when it comes to hugs. Taps on the shoulder are often a good starting point.
- Be extremely careful about touching at work. Some workplaces are hypersensitive about touching. Make your touches in the office feel friendly, not flirty.

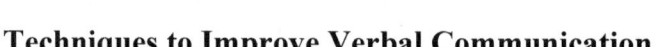

One Step at a Time

– Give directions in step-wise format
  - Avoid "first we will..then we will...then.."
  - Keep them concrete
  - Asking someone to "stand up, pick up the mallet, then sit back down" may be too much
  - One instruction at a time
  - Don't have to be verbal

Techniques to Improve Verbal Communication

- **Talk to the person in a non-distracting place.** A person with dementia cannot concentrate amid environmental distractions such as competing conversations or background television noise.
- **Start conversations with orientation.** Identify yourself and use their name.
- **Use short words and short, simple sentences.**
- **Speak slowly and say individual words clearly.**
- ***But* do not talk down to the person with dementia.** Speak as to any adult friend. Show respect.
- **Use a low tone (pitch) of voice.** A raised pitch is a signal that one is upset. A person with a hearing impairment is also able to hear a lower pitch more readily.
- **Speak to the person with dementia in a warm, easy-going, and pleasant manner.** Use non-verbal clues, including facial expressions, tone of voice, or touch to show your feelings of affection. Smiling, taking the person's hand, or touching the person's arm, can vividly communicate that you are interested and really care.

- **Take your time when giving instructions.** Allow plenty of time for the information to be absorbed. Give the person plenty of time to respond. What seems like unproductive silence may actually be hardworking concentration for the person with dementia.
- **Give clear and simple instructions.** If you repeat an instruction, repeat it exactly. If the person does not seem to understand, try other ways of saying it.
- **Ask the person to do one thing at a time.** He/she is probably incapable of remembering a series of instructions. Daily living activities involve several tasks such as getting dressed, taking a bath, or sitting down in a chair or wheelchair. Break each activity down into a number of small steps. This is called task-breakdown. It is important that the breakdown of steps be adapted to each person's ability.

Source: (Veterans Affairs Canada)
There is an endless variety of factors which act as roadblocks or barriers to effective communication. We will look at some of the factors which may affect the quality of a message:
1. **Past Experience**: If your relationship has a history of poor communicating, it takes a major effort to lift this roadblock. People often respond out of habit - a conditioned or learned response. Example: People who moan and groan and complain frequently can find that even their valid complaints may be overlooked. Conversely, the person who consistently puts on a brave face may be viewed as "getting along just fine" when, in fact, they are hiding a lot of distress.
2. **Mood**: Any mood, from "good" to "bad" and including a range of emotions, can affect our interpretation of messages. A mood may be temporary and often responds to subtle overtones.
3. **Personalities**: Each personality is unique; sometimes we just need to accept people as they are.
4. **Perceptions**: Perceptions arise from attitudes, feelings, knowledge and past experiences. Perceptions affect the way

we interact with each other. It is said that perception is reality. People respond and/or behave with feelings appropriate to their perceptions. If the perceptions are based on faulty information, the feelings may be viewed by others as inappropriate.

Empathy, putting oneself in another's shoes, is an essential quality to improve communication. Challenge yourself: the next time you are in a situation where you feel the person is responding inappropriately, stop and ask yourself what might their perceptions be?

5. **Self-image**: A poor self-image affects all aspects of your persona. It may drastically alter an individual's capacity to communicate with others; there may be no energy for empathy, sharing or reaching out.

   A poor self-image may lead a person to be misjudged. Several aspects affect our self-esteem, including health, feedback from other people, achievement, finances, and opportunities to be useful. The care receiver and caregiver may experience losses in these areas which leave them feeling very vulnerable.

6. **Distraction**: There could be a fear of being overheard or perhaps excessive background activity or noise affecting the quality of communication.

7. **Sensory Deficits**: We will discuss sensory losses in detail a bit later. Decrease in sensory acuity is a normal part of aging. A loss such as reduced hearing can have a profound effect on communication.

Listening Skills

- Listening is probably the most important communication skill we can acquire.
- Good listening requires empathy, attention and valid feedback.
- There are many benefits to listening: people feel valued and cared for.
- When you listen effectively, you do not necessarily need to agree with the other person, but you do need to convey interest (respect and empathy).

- Do not interrupt, especially to correct mistakes. It is important to accept and understand the uniqueness of the speaker's feelings and perspective.
- One technique for good listening is reflecting the feelings that the other person has shared (follow your instincts).This can involve both paraphrasing (clarifying what the messages mean to you) and perception-checking (describing your impressions of another's feelings).

Dementia
- There are many causes for symptoms of dementia; some are reversible, some are not. Dementia such as the Alzheimer type develops gradually over time. If there are symptoms of intellectual decline in someone you know, it is always important to speak to a medical professional.
- When dementia is present, there can be great fluctuation in abilities from day to day. Sometimes it is difficult to know what to expect and how to respond.

Note: If the person you are caring for suddenly becomes quite confused, you should always notify the doctor. This can be an indication of an illness.

Some communication problems associated with dementia include:
1. difficulty in expressing oneself to others
2. problems in understanding what others say
- It is important to remember that feelings usually remain intact in the memory-impaired person. Even if a person cannot communicate verbally, he or she can often still relate on a "feelings" level.
- It is a challenge to communicate without "talking down" to the person. The following suggestions are adapted from Facilitating Communication with the Frail Elderly. Roberta Way-Clark, 1990.
- Techniques to Aid Communication with a Person Suffering from Dementia:
  - Reflect back content and feelings to determine meaning.
  - Ask simple questions; be clear and direct.
  - Give clear, simple instructions, one task at a time.
  - Talk to the person in a non-distracting place.

- Begin conversation with orienting information.
- Call the person with dementia by name.
- Explain the purpose of your visit.
- Use short words and simple sentences but avoid "talking down"; the person can sense this.
- Treat people with the respect and dignity you would wish to have.
- Speak slowly and say individual words clearly.
- Lower the pitch of your voice; a raised pitch indicates you are upset.
- Use non-verbal cues like touch and facial expression, i.e., smiling.

There are two other techniques that should be mentioned:

Reality Orientation. The speaker provides information about name, location, date, daily events, etc. verbally or on strategically placed display boards. Environmental aids are used: large calendar, clocks, display boards, tags, etc.

Validation Therapy. This approach accepts the validity of the old, frail person who has returned to the past. It accepts memories as important components of a person's life in order to understand their motivation and behaviour in the present. It validates feelings generated by loss.

Example: You are caring for your mother, who suffers from dementia. She informs you that her mother is coming to visit this afternoon. How would you respond?

1. Mom, you know that your mother is dead (said kindly).
2. Mom, tell me about your mother. What was she like? (Validation Therapy)

Affirmation, Flexibility & Fun

- Lots of Praise or Acknowledgment
  - Should respect their adulthood
- Be Flexible
  - Agitation and wandering
- Have Fun!
  - Remember pace

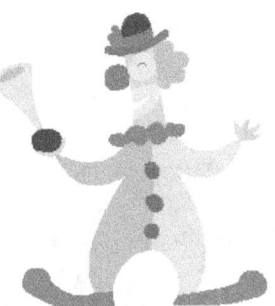

Source: (South Lakes Alzheimer's Disease Society)

Problems in communicating with a person who has dementia often arise because of our own expectations of the person. Frequently, someone who is very close to the person with dementia feels that he/she is purposefully being difficult.

The environment and the use of nonverbal communication (Body Language) are very important in communicating. Avoid a noisy or hectic environment. Be alert to any changes in the person's environment. If he/she seems to be disturbed, move him/her to a quieter environment. Many people with Alzheimer's are keenly aware of the emotional climate.

Body language is a very important tool when working with a person who has dementia. Never approach the person quickly from behind. Approach calmly from the side at an angle or from the front, saying his/her name. Make certain that your body is saying what your voice and words are saying. Do not move too quickly and do not appear too hurried.

Touch the person or use some sort of visual aid. Use simple sentences. Say, "Time for a bath," instead of, "Hello, how are you? It's time for your bath now."

If the person does not respond after a wait, repeat the question with gestures. If you say "Stop that!" or "Not now!" in a sharp tone, the person will probably respond in a similar manner. Moderate your tone and words.

Determine what the person is trying to communicate. If the person is restless or agitated, do not force communication.

Watch the person's eyes and body language. They may show fear, pain, or anger. If the person does not want to talk to you, he/she will avoid eye contact; fold his/her arms and/or fidget. When the person wishes to communicate he/she will often smile, appear to be relaxed, lean closer to you, and/or touch you. When the person rambles and seems to be making no sense, try to listen to "key" words. Often a few blurted words reveal the true message he/she is attempting to communicate.

Sensations from the skin are represented by a large area of the brain and therefore stand more chance of "getting through" to someone with Alzheimer's disease. Communication with gentle touch reduces feelings of confusion and rejection and increases mutual understanding.

Individuals suffering from a dementia have difficulty understanding what is told to them. Often questions and instructions have no meaning. The caregiver or family member may misinterpret responses or lack of response as uncooperative or inattentive behavior.

Some people with dementia cannot communicate a whole thought, but can express a few words of the thought. Some may understand you, but are unable to form an answer. As the dementia increases, some may repeat a phrase or a series of rhyming words. However, some of these sounds have meaning to the person uttering them.

Summary

- Be aware of their needs
- Goal is:
  - Their understanding, not
  - Your deliverance
- Relax, give them space and time
- Use humor and touch when appropriate
- Be flexible and affirming

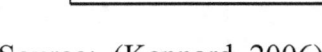

Source: (Kennard, 2006)

Tips for Effective Communication

- When someone has Alzheimer's disease, or any other form of dementia, communication can become more difficult. Their understanding of what you are saying and their ability to make you understand their world can be highly variable and each person will react to different stimuli in different ways. This means we have to be sensitive to the way we present ourselves and how we give information when we talk with someone with Alzheimer's or other forms of dementia.
- For the most effective way to talk and communicate with someone who has Alzheimer's it is important to remember a few simple rules
- Body language, communication and Alzheimer's
- Your facial expression, your body language, the tone of your voice become extra important when talking and communicating to someone with neurological problems. If a person with dementia feels threatened, undermined or confused by your communication with them they may react in a negative way to your interventions i.e. conversation or information can increase agitation, undermine their confidence, increase their feelings of isolation.

Environmental Awareness Aids Communication

- Is the lighting sufficient to aid communication? In conversation we usually look at the face and body of the person talking to us. It helps us to understand content and intent. Make sure you have some light on your face.
- Identify yourself and address the person by name.
- This helps someone with Alzheimer's to orientate.
- Does the person with dementia have hearing or sight difficulties?
- Make allowances for visual and hearing deficits. Look into getting a medical evaluation and aids to assist communication.
- Make sure you have the person's attention.
- Speak slowly, calmly and distinctly.
- For effective communication you need to balance distinctive speech without treating the person with dementia as a child, without shouting or becoming angry with them if they do not understand. Shouting also affects the tone of your voice and makes understanding more difficult. Do not get angry even if you find yourself becoming frustrated. We will all have seen people talking too loudly at people with dementia, it is not nice, and it really does not help their self respect and confidence.
- Use simple, direct statements and information.
- Use words the person can understand.
- Do not give more than one instruction at a time.
- Do not press for an answer if that worries or confuses them.
- Ask questions that require a "yes" or "no" response if that aids conversation and understanding.
- If you do not understand the content of their conversation.
- If you do not understand what they have said you can ask them to repeat it. Sometimes conversing with someone with Alzheimer's is not necessarily about understanding; it is about showing care, concern, inclusion, and love towards them.
- Correcting wrong information.

- It is not necessary to constantly correct the validity of the person's statements if it includes wrong information.
- Give visual cues and write things down.
- Minimize distracting noise.
- If your conversation has not been successful try again later.

Works Cited

Cummings, T. (n.d.). *Seven Steps to Communicating With Dementia Adults*. Retrieved Nov 2010, from Area Agency on Aging: http://www.aaacap.org/Cummings%20Seven%20Steps%20to%20Communicating%20With%20Dementia%20Adults.pdf

Dobson, R. (2006, Oct 11). *How the power of touch reduces pain and even fights disease*. Retrieved Apr 2010, from The Independent: http://www.independent.co.uk/life-style/health-and-families/health-news/how-the-power-of-touch-reduces-pain-and-even-fights-disease-419462.html

Kennard, C. (2006, June 22). *Talking to People with Dementia*. Retrieved Oct 2010, from Alzheimer's Disease: http://alzheimers.about.com/od/frustration/a/talking_dementi.htm

Science Daily. (n.d.). *Happiness Is 'Infectious' In Network Of Friends: Collective -- Not Just Individual -- Phenomenon*. Retrieved Oct 2010, from Science Daily: http://www.sciencedaily.com/releases/2008/12/081205094506.htm

South Lakes Alzheimer's Disease Society. (n.d.). *Additional strategies for communicating with a person who has dementia*. Retrieved Mar 2010, from Alzheimer's Disease Society: http://easyweb.easynet.co.uk/vob/alzheimers/information/Communicat.htm

Veterans Affairs Canada. (n.d.). *Communication Skills for Caregivers*. Retrieved Oct 2010, from Veterans Affairs Canada: http://www.vac-acc.gc.ca/providers/sub.cfm?source=caregivrmanual/sect4/module3/workshop3

Chapter 8 - Environmental & Structural Accommodations and Safety

---

1. Accommodations

- People with dementia often have more difficulty perceiving depth, discriminating among colors, or seeing contrast.

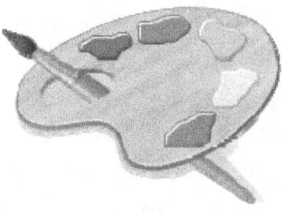

Source: (Canadian Psychological Association)

In addition to the changes in vision or hearing that come with aging, people with dementia often have more difficulty perceiving depth, discriminating among colors, or seeing contrast. Some changes to the home environment may help the person manage these difficulties.

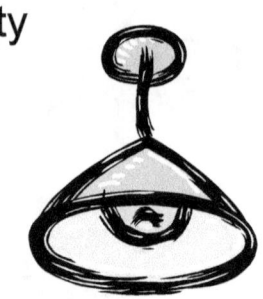

2. Safety

- Eliminating clutter
- Install railings
- Increase lighting
- Reduce glare
- Color code rooms
- Hang a curtain over locked doors

Source: (Canadian Psychological Association)

- Eliminating confusing clutter or unneeded furniture that hinders easy movement.
- Installing railings on stairs to reduce falls.
- Increasing lighting in active areas of the home, particularly stairways.
- Reducing glare (i.e., non-glare flooring, adjustable window blinds).
- Color-coding rooms.
- In the event that a door must remain locked to prevent the person from exiting unsafely, it may help to hang a curtain over the locked door that is the same color as the surrounding walls. In this way, the door is less noticeable so the risk of exit can be lessened.

Adapting a home for a person with dementia requires changes to the physical space as well as changes to activities and the ways in which we interact with the person. To create an environment that is as safe and pleasant as possible, we need to take into account any behavioral problems the person might experience as well as his or her likes, dislikes and habits.

1. Sensory sensitivity and visuospatial abilities

In addition to the changes in vision or hearing that come with aging, people with dementia often have more difficulty perceiving depth, discriminating among colors, or seeing contrast. Some changes to the home environment may help the person manage these difficulties. They include: eliminating confusing clutter or unneeded furniture that hinder easy movement; installing railings on stairs to reduce falls; increasing lighting in active areas of the home, particularly stairways; reducing glare (i.e., non-glare flooring, adjustable window blinds); color-coding rooms; and in the event that a door must remain locked to prevent the person from exiting unsafely, it may help to hang a curtain over the locked door that is the same color as the surrounding walls. In this way, the door is less noticeable so the risk of exit can be lessened.

2. Memory and other cognitive functions

 Memory and cognitive functions enable us to find our way in the environment, know the time, date and where we are, and carry on conversations, etc.

For the person with dementia, losses in these functions can lead to confusion, agitation and a loss of independence and control over the environment.

There are strategies and cues we can use to help the person with dementia better accomplish some of these activities, maintain some independence and control over the environment and reduce the need for him or her to repetitively ask for missing information. These include: the use of labels or pictures on cupboards to show content (e.g., coffee cup); pasting familiar signs or images on doors to identify room function (e.g., toilet sign, picture of a bed); creating a "memory box" that contains small personal items that can trigger meaningful conversation (e.g., pictures of family members, pets or possessions); setting and maintaining the same daily schedule to provide a sense of control over the environment; posting the schedule on a picture board may also reduce often repeated questions;

prominently displaying clocks and calendars; posting a list of favorite television programs with their times and channels near the TV to increase autonomy and decrease repetitive questions; setting-up computer function keys, with meaningful stick-on labels, to facilitate easy Internet and e-mail connections; and using Velcro fasteners on clothing instead of buttons.

3.   Behavior

Behavioral problems are a major cause of stress and safety concern for persons with dementia and their caregivers. They are also the number one reason why persons with dementia are cared for in institutions.

Behavioral problems include agitation, aggression, repetitive questioning, and wandering unsafely. Feelings of frustration, confusion, insecurity, boredom, and feeling overwhelmed can underlie behavioral problems.

There are a number of environmental adaptations that can successfully reduce or eliminate some of these behaviors.

a)   Verbally Agitated and Aggressive Behavior.

Angry and hostile outbursts, verbal harassment, screaming, cursing, or using obscene and/or profane language are the most common kinds of behavioral problems in persons with dementia.

Such behavior can result from frustration due to difficulty communicating or understanding what is being said, feeling overwhelmed by too much information or too much noise (particularly at sundown), trying to do a task that is too difficult, uncertainty or fear that comes from the lack of control over the environment, or even boredom, fatigue or hunger.

Environmental adaptations that can help include: using picture boards that encourage pointing at pictures to express needs; using computers as a two-way communication aid; simplifying instructions; reducing noise or other stimulation; designating a room as a quiet place for retreat; playing soft music; following a routine to decrease uncertainty;

and providing cues to help with transitions (e.g., smell of cooking helps prepare for meal time, bringing out a lap blanket can signal rest or quiet time).

b)   Physically Agitated and Aggressive Behavior.

Although far less common, these behaviors are highly stressful for the caregiver. They include assault or violent behavior, throwing objects, hitting, kicking, biting, hair pulling, pushing, scratching, tearing things, damaging property and/or making threatening gestures.

Physical aggression may result from the same kinds of difficulties and feelings that underlie verbal aggression. They include over-stimulation, feeling overwhelmed if a task is too difficult, or not recognizing someone or something the person is being asked to recognize.

The environmental adaptations listed under verbally aggressive behavior may be of help here as well, particularly the use of a quiet room as well as simplifying tasks and instructions.

c)   Verbally Agitated and Non-Aggressive Behavior.

These include such behaviors as repeating sentences or questions, making strange noises, muttering, complaining or being negative and frequent requests for attention – all of which can be irritating and stressful for the caregiver. These behaviors often reflect a need for reassurance.

Provide reassurance – particularly if the person can no longer recognize you; play soft music in the background; introduce a familiar physical object or activity; post a daily schedule, and point to it when moving to the next item on the agenda; adhere to the schedule; use timers to remind the person of plans or activities; and try some of the adaptations suggested above under the section titled Memory and other cognitive functions.

d)   Physically Agitated and Non-Aggressive Behavior.

These behaviors are less frequent in persons with dementia and include wandering, pacing aimlessly, elopement, inappropriately following people, hyperactivity, robing or disrobing, repetitive mannerisms or actions, and restlessness. They can result from boredom, under-stimulation, or a need to feel useful.

Provide new or more activities and things to do; increase the variety of activities provided to include the different senses (e.g., particularly things that can be touched); provide opportunities for more involvement in day-to-day activities (e.g., safe aspects of meal preparation, clean-up); and provide more social opportunities.

Short videos on this topic, demonstrating solutions to problems such as repetitive behaviors or difficult behaviors, can be viewed at: http://www.theonlinequilt.com.

4.   Personal preferences and habits.

In order to enhance quality of life and reduce problem behaviors that can occur in dementia, it is important to find the right balance of environmental stimulation and support.

For example, people who are under-stimulated may feel bored and restless. On the other hand, people who are over-stimulated may feel overwhelmed and can act out. The environment should be carefully adapted to the changes and losses faced by the person with dementia while preserving the memories, experiences, interests and habits unique to that person.

1. Accommodations

- Bathroom – safety locks on cabinets containing household cleaning agents

- Kitchen – safety locks on drawers & cabinets containing matches, liquor, knives, cleaning agents

- Stove – safety knobs & timers

In the bathroom, install safety locks on cabinets containing medicines, household cleaning agents, razors and other potentially dangerous items. You can also move these items to a padlocked toolbox or elsewhere.

In the kitchen, put safety locks on drawers or cabinets containing matches, liquor, knives, household cleaning agents, scissors, and any other potentially dangerous items.

Put safety knobs on your stove, or install a timer so the stove can only operate during certain hours.

1. Accommodations

- Lower water heater temperature to 120

- Remove locks from bathroom & bedroom doors

- Additional locks on exterior doors

- Swimming pool fence or firm cover

Lower the temperature on the water heater to 120 degrees and label all hot-water faucets clearly with large, red letters. All seniors are at greater risk for scalding because of thinner skin and slower reaction times, and a person with dementia who may not recognize the danger even more so.

Remove locks from bathroom and bedroom doors. A senior with Alzheimer's might lock a door and then not remember how to unlock it.

Place additional locks on doors a senior might use to leave the house and wander off. Locate the locks high up on the door or somewhere else difficult for the senior to find.

If you have a swimming pool, take precautions to prevent the senior from falling or wading in. Install a firm pool cover or put up a fence with a locked gate.

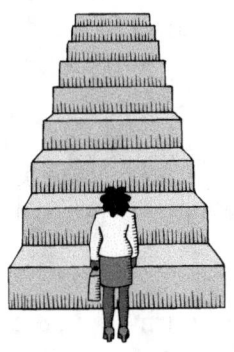

2. Safety

- Remove clutter – obstacles

- Decorate with solid colors

- Keep home well-light at night

- Stay calm and respond softly

Source: (U.S. Department of Health and Human Services)
Remove all clutter, throw rugs, and other potential obstacles. Make sure hallways are clear and easy to navigate.

Decorate with solid colors whenever possible. Patterns can confuse someone with Alzheimer's.

Keep the home well-lighted at night. Waking up in total darkness can disorient an Alzheimer's patient.

Reduce clutter in the room and bathroom
- Take home items no longer needed by the resident.
- Keep pathways clear at all times.
- Watch for telephone and electrical cords in the walking area.
- Keep the over bed table across the bed.
- Make sure that the furniture you bring is stable and doesn't tilt if the resident leans on it. Don't bring in cardboard furniture, pedestal tables or tables with three legs. When you leave the room, take a quick look around. Do you see any clutter, cords, furniture or other items in pathways? Remove items or call for help from staff. Make sure the call light and personal items are within easy reach of the resident when you leave.

Safe shoes and slippers
- All shoes and slippers should fit well and have a firm shape. Shoes should have a low, even heel. While some carpets may cause problems for residents who wear shoes with deep tread, generally speaking, all shoes and slippers should have some form of tread on the sole. Examples include tennis shoes with Velcro fasteners, oxford style shoes and canvas or leather slip-on shoes.
- If a resident cannot wear safe shoes or slippers, use gripper socks instead.
- Use gripper socks at night.

Safety during transfer and bathroom use
- Always call for help from staff when you are unsure about helping your family member get out of bed or go to the bathroom. Do not transfer an unsteady resident alone.
- Bring in easy-to-manage clothing such as pants with elastic bands, easy to pull up skirts and dresses, and items with Velcro fasteners.
- Lock wheelchair brakes before transfer.
- Use all prescribed seating items for a resident when she is in the wheelchair.

Help the patient to use low blood pressure precautions
- Before the resident gets out of bed, ask her to sit on the edge and dangle her feet for a few minutes.
- Encourage the resident to flex her feet backwards several times while sitting.
- Remind the resident not to tilt her head backwards.
- After meals and anytime the resident has been sitting for a while, encourage her to get up slowly and to use assistance. Report any complaints of dizziness.

Reducing Falls: A Safety Checklist for the Home

Accidents in the home are a major cause of injury. One in three people 65 years and older fall every year and most of these falls happen in the home. This checklist helps to identify safety problems and provides easy tips for making your home a safer place. Use your common sense and take action to correct the problems you find. Most solutions are not expensive. If you cannot fix the problem yourself, ask a family member or friend to help.

Put a check beside each safety problem you find in your home. Then read the suggestions for improving the problem.

Do you have:

___ Unsafe stairs? Broken or worn stairs?

Repair broken or worn steps. Edges of stairs should be clearly visible with coverings in good condition and securely fastened down. Never store items on steps. Keep them free of clutter.

___ Broken or missing railings?

Porch and stair railings should be checked regularly. Make certain they are secure. Repair or install handrails on both sides of the stairs. Handrails should continue for the entire length of the staircase.

___ Poor lighting around stairs or dark hallways?

Increase the wattage of bulbs to the maximum allowed by the fixture. Add illuminated light switch plates to make it easy to find switches in the dark. Make sure that light switches are located at both the top and bottom of stairways. Add bright strips of tape to the edge of each stair.

___ Throw rugs?

Either remove them or fasten them securely to the floor with adhesive, double-stick tape. Do not use loose rugs anywhere, especially at the bottom of stairs.

__ Clutter?

Keep pathways clear. Put away shoes, newspapers, books, and other items and keep them off the floor. Make sure that electrical and telephone cords are not in pathways. Keep cords out from underneath carpet. Coil or attach cords to the baseboard. Have an electrician add another outlet if needed. Arrange furniture in order to give plenty of walking room.

__ Hard to reach items?

Cabinets and closets often have shelves that are too high to reach safely. Store frequently used items on the lowest shelf, at waist level. Avoid using stools and never stand on a chair to reach high items. If you do use a stool, use a steady step stool with a bar for support. Use a long-handled grasper to reach high objects.

__ A slippery bathroom floor, bathtub or shower?

Use a non-skid mat in the shower and bathtub. Use a rubber mat or nonskid strips in front of the sink, bathtub and shower to avoid slipping on wet spots. If you bathe in a shower, consider installing a non-skid shower chair and hand-held shower head so you can sit while bathing.

Avoid pulling up on the sink, a towel rack or soap dish to get up from the toilet or bathtub. These are not intended to support your weight and may come off the wall. Install grab bars or handrails in the shower, on walls around the bathtub, and beside the toilet. Make sure they are securely fastened to the wall to support your weight. There are specially designed commode chairs that can improve safety as well.

__ Not enough lighting? Too much glare?

Use maximum wattage bulbs allowed by each fixture. Use lights that shine directly on your work area for specific tasks. Use frosted bulbs, globes and shades on fixtures to reduce glare. Avoid shiny surfaces that may increase glare. If overhead lighting is not enough, add lamps. Consider installing motion detector lights that turn on automatically.

Install easy-access light switches at the entrance to a room so you do not have to walk in the dark in order to turn on the light.

Always use a night light in the bathroom. Use a night light that automatically turns on in low-light situations. Make sure that you can light the path from your bed to the bathroom easily while en route. Keep a flashlight by your bed.

Make sure there is adequate lighting outside by walkways and entrances. Use a motion sensor light that will turn on whenever there is movement.

__ Furniture that is difficult to get out of?

Sit on furniture that has good back support. Firm chairs with sturdy armrests provide more support when rising. Add pillows to the back of the chair so that your feet rest firmly on the floor.

__ Unstable furniture?

Use tables that have four legs. Do not use tripod or pedestal tables. Repair the legs or add stabilizers to furniture that rocks or tilts when you lean on it.

__ Loose carpet or linoleum?

Tack down loose carpeting everywhere in your home, especially on stairs. Make sure that there are no curled or frayed edges. Replace missing linoleum or any tile that is broken or loose.

__ Spills or wet spots?

Wipe up spills immediately. Clean up any liquid, grease, or food spilled on the floor.

__ Gutters or windows that need to be cleaned?

If you use a stepladder, make sure someone is bracing it for you. Don't overextend your reach.

__ Cracks or uneven places in cement walks or stairways? Slippery pavement?

Patch cracks with filler before they spread. Avoid broken sidewalks. Be very careful on wet or icy pavement. Make sure your walkways are shoveled and cleared of ice and snow in the winter. Use salt or an ice-melting product to keep surfaces clear of ice.

__ Pets?

Don't let a pet catch you by surprise by running through your feet. Always be aware of your pet's location.

When someone in your home uses a wheelchair, there are many things that can be done to improve access. Narrow doors can be enlarged and heavy or hard-to-open doors can be altered. Ramps can be added to entrances. Changes in the kitchen and bathroom can be made to accommodate wheelchairs as well.

This brochure does not include all potential causes of falls. It is not intended as medical advice and should not be a substitute for professional advice from your health care provider. Contact your doctor or health care provider if you have questions or need help making changes. Remember to keep a phone with emergency numbers within easy reach.

References:
The Fall Prevention Project, Southeast Senior Housing Initiative, Baltimore, MD, 1997.
Safe at Home, Magee Rehabilitation Jefferson Health System, Philadelphia, PA, 2002.
Home Solutions, American Association of Retired Persons, Washington, DC, 1999.
Home Care of the Elderly, Sheryl Zang and Judith Allender, Philadelphia, PA, 1999.
Home Safety Checklist, American Academy of Orthopaedic Surgeons, Des Plaines, Illinois, 2000.
Check for Safety, Centers for Disease Control, Atlanta, Georgia, 1999.

2. Safety

- Solid black mats in front of doors leading outside

- Constantly check inside and out for potentially dangerous items

- Maintain routine, provide advance notice to change

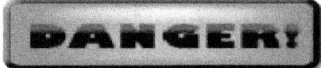

Place solid black mats on the floor in front of doors leading outside. These can appear as deep holes to an Alzheimer's patient and may keep them from passing through the door.

Check outside the house for potentially dangerous items such as saws, lighter fluid, power tools, and paint. Put such items in a locked garage or tool shed.

Summary

- Lower the clutter, decrease the furniture

- Use solid simple patterns for cloth

- Safety locks on cabinetry

- Continuously search for dangerous objects

Source: (Rice)

Home Safety and Dementia

By Karen L. Rice, M.A., LNHA
Gerontologist, Negotiator, Mediator

The cognitive problems that a person with dementia experiences
because a variety of home safety concerns. This is an ongoing concern
for family members, because as the individual's dementia progresses,
so do the needs for care. You should continually evaluate the ability
of your parent to live at home safely. Questions to regularly ask are:

- Can the elder recognize a dangerous situation, like a fire?
- Does the elder know how to use the telephone for getting help?
- How content is he or she at home?
- Are there signs of agitation, depression, or withdrawal?
- Does the elder wander?
- Is his or her confusion increasing?

The more the answers to these questions spell risk, the more you
should consider placement in a specialized long-term care facility to
reduce the chance of danger.

Kitchen - Simple steps like unplugging appliances can eliminate a
potential danger. Inserting plastic outlet covers makes it more difficult
for the elder to plug the appliance back in. Faucets can be restricted
with heavy rubber bands. Remove equipment like knives, can
openers, matches, chemicals and decorative items like throw rugs.
Install inside locks (e.g., child safety locks) on drawers and cabinets.
Locks on outside doors will keep the elder safely inside the house.

Bathroom - Medicine, razors, soaps and chemicals should be stored
and locked in one place. Color-code or label faucets "hot" and "cold."
In the tub/shower area, grab bars, nonskid mats, and shower chairs are
helpful. Consider posting reminders in the bathroom (such as
"FLUSH TOILET" or "EXIT") and elsewhere around the house.

Living and Dining Rooms - Simplify the layout of rooms by
rearranging furniture. Remove light-weight furniture that a confused
elder could move easily. Eliminate obstacles like cords, throw rugs,

and knickknacks so that the senior can move about freely. It is important to keep the environment (here and elsewhere in the house) uncluttered to reduce confusion and agitation.

Halls and Stairways - Address a demented elder's impaired senses by installing smoke alarms in case he cannot smell smoke himself. Nightlights can help guide the elder. Similarly, dark areas warn him where not to go. In some cases, darkness can "erase" a room or hallway in the mind of a demented person. Darkening areas is one way of detouring a wandering elder. Add color contrast at the edges of stairs to help the elder differentiate between steps.

Works Cited

Canadian Psychological Association. (n.d.). *ENVIRONMENTAL ADAPTATIONS TO DEMENTIA*. Retrieved Apr 2009, from http://www.cpa.ca/publications/yourhealthpsychologyworksfac tsheets/environmentaladaptationstodementia/

Rice, K. (n.d.). *Home Safety and Dementia*. Retrieved Oct 2010, from Care Minds: Sharing the Wisdom of Elder Care: http://www.careminds.com/article/show/18

U.S. Department of Health and Human Services. (n.d.). *Ways Families Can Help Reduce Fall Risk*. Retrieved Oct 2010, from http://www.ahrq.gov/research/ltc/fallspx/fallspxmanapb8.htm